COMPENDIUM OF VIRTUAL & TRADITIONAL FITNESS

A Comprehensive Fitness and Wellness Guide
for Instructors, Trainers, Therapists,
Virtual Trainers, Fitness Enthusiasts
and Participants . . . *EVERYONE!*

MARC D. THOMPSON

Illustrations and Photographs
by Dana Donaty

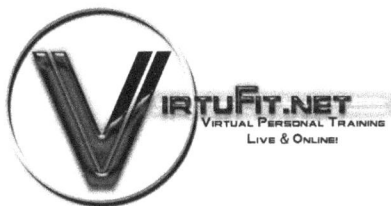

VirtuFit.NET
VIRTUAL PERSONAL TRAINING
LIVE & ONLINE!

Disclaimer: This book is offered as information to guide your research to better health. All statements, suggestions, content has not been evaluated by any governing body of any country and is only to offer general knowledge to help individuals or health care providers to develop the best life possible. This book and website and any other product, person, institution, business or otherwise is not intended to diagnose, prevent or cure any disease, physically or mentally and is also not intended to provide any legal, financial, spiritual or religious advice. This book, website and anything and anyone else related to this book and website, do not accept responsibility for any liability, harm, loss, damage or any other reactions to, or for any use of, the information offered. Please consult your health practitioners before beginning any fitness regimen.

MARC D. THOMPSON, VIRTUFIT®

Online Skype Personal Training, Live & Online!

www.VirtuFit.net • marc@VirtuFit.net

skype: VirtuFit

Produced by The Book Couple • www.thebookcouple.com

Contents

CHAPTER 2. MUSCULAR & RESISTANCE WORKOUTS

CHAPTER 3. REHABILITATION & RECOVERY WORKOUTS

CHAPTER 4. PILATES & YOGA WORKOUTS

CHAPTER 5. FLEXIBILITY & BALANCE WORKOUTS

CHAPTER 6. VIRTUAL WORKOUTS & ONLINE FITNESS

CHAPTER 7. GENERAL FITNESS & SAFETY

Chapter 8. Nutrition & Mindfulness

Chapter 9. Fitness Quotes & Proverbs

ACKNOWLEDGEMENTS

Many, many thanks to every client I have had over the past thirty years. You have allowed me to experience the truth of wellness. Thank you also to my mentors who have molded and educated me along the way, especially my mother, Shirley, my first coach, Sarah Johnson and my grandfather, Harper Thompson.

Dedicated to ye who reads this book
and seeks the wisdom of being fit
in mind, body and spirit

Preface

by Annette Annechild, PhD

It is with great pleasure that I introduce you to the inimitable Marc D. Thompson and his *Compendium of Virtual & Traditional Fitness.* What makes this book so special is that it is perfect for the beginner, as well as for the seasoned professional. What makes the lists themselves so special is they have captured both the art and science of Marc's decades of experience in the fitness field.

Marc approaches fitness with the same positivity with which he approaches life. Wherever your journey has taken your body up to this point, this book can take you to the next step. I know that for certain, because he has taken me there. I have been in the fitness world for decades myself. I have seven books out in the field and years of training under my belt. I was a competitive bodybuilder and have been a yoga teacher for over twenty years. Then, I met Marc.

In some ways, my fitness journey started over there. Marc is focused on all aspects of fitness. Way beyond the mirror, he has knowledge in all aspects of a truly fit body. I had thought I was fit but in reality I wasn't nearly as conditioned as I became with Marc. My balance, endurance, and form vastly improved.

This book can teach you to stretch correctly, eat well, condition your heart, and tone every muscle of your body. Beyond fitness fads, there are truths about training and you now hold all of them in your hands. My advice is read it from cover to cover. Then, make a plan. Choose from the lists and jump right in. I have always been impressed that working with Marc's lists seemed so manageable, almost too easy to produce such impressive results. But they do, and they will for you. Just turn the page and get going; you are going to love where this book takes you.

Foreword

Marc Thompson's diverse and unique ways of teaching and helping others to improve their physical appearance and conditions are very inspiring and effective. Marc's different approaches to physical wellness are the product of many years of experience and professionalism at what he enjoys doing the best. Life can be busy, stressful, and even unfair, however we always have the inner power to learn and develop the healthiest lifestyles or to reach out for help to someone like Marc to guide us finding new methods to aim at and achieve those desired results. This *Compendium of Virtual & Traditional Fitness* is a necessary and valuable addition to everyone's book shelf.

—Antonella Martino, PharmD

I have been a primary healthcare provider for over twenty years, during which time I have developed the ability to recognize something useful and effective that can lead to positive results for a client's physical health and personal well-being. Marc Thompson's *Compendium of Virtual & Traditional Fitness* is just that and more. Marc is a master trainer whose unique enthusiasm, vast knowledge, and excellent techniques fill the pages of his new training manual.

Delivered in a style which is innovative and truly cutting-edge, revealing his experience, his positive attitude, and his great affinity for people, Marc's formula for attaining higher levels of health through proper training exposes his purpose—to reach as many people as possible and to change their existence, helping them to have healthier, happier lives.

I am proud to be Marc Thompson's friend and professional colleague; he is doing something positive about today's illnesses and suffering. We could all use this kind of "how-to" manual in our quest for optimal physical health, and Marc has given us a great resource. Get this manual and change your life and the lives of your friends and loved ones.

—Edward M. Scarlett, LicAc, DiplAc

Introduction

I THINK IN LISTS. One of my first experiences with lists came after I graduated from college. For nine years, I kept a daily list of everything related to my health and fitness. My lists included what I ate, when I ate it, how I exercised, what type of exercise I engaged in, my energy level, my sleep routine, how I felt, and my frame of mind. By the end of nine years, I knew exactly what I had to do to feel good, stay in shape and be healthy.

A second experience occurred at a well-known gym. I was a new trainer and decided my job would be simplified if I could come up with a comprehensive list of all the exercises I might use to help each client. I pulled out a pen and notebook and started with free weights. Within about 20 minutes I had listed 1,000 exercises in my notebook. The following week I counted 600 free-weight exercises on my list. I realized I hadn't even touched machines, med balls, bands, etc. Something was wrong with my list.

Third, I realized the need for virtual webcam training. I independently developed a complete live webcam personal training and yoga business in 2008. I learned from trial and error the ways to keep clients healthy from distances as far away as New Delhi, Ireland, and Canada.

Lastly, I noticed how much faster my clients progressed if we combined cognitive, spiritual and physical exercises together. The holistic training led to improvements that separately was not possible.

These discoveries and others transformed my philosophy of fitness. I realized there are an exhaustive number of exercises for each muscle, but only a limited number of movements each muscle can make. With a simple, structured, foundation based on kinesiology, I began to analyze a client's needs and limitations creatively. I introduced a variety of tools, classes, and pieces of equipment to move and build each muscle without injury, propelling the client toward his or her goals. Not only does this method limit injury and build muscles, it makes exercising fun and dynamic.

Wellness is certainly not an absolute and often a case when less is more. Both student and teacher alike, must take each list not literally but more creatively. Use these fundamentals and adapt them to suit you and your clientele in a healthy, meaningful way.

Overall, my hope in putting these lists together is to make readers, including participants, fitness professionals and health care workers, aware of the importance of variety in wellness prescription so as to avoid injury, impart maximum benefits, and make exercise fun and interesting. I also want every reader to have an easy resource to build personal, flexible exercise programs. We've added hundreds of more exercises, three major categories, detailed the VPT training portion and we've included Humorous Proverbs and Client Quotes.

CHAPTER 1

Warmup & Cardiovascular Workouts

CARDIOVASCULAR TRAINING. Physical conditioning that strengthens heart and blood vessels, the result of which is an increase in the ability for your body muscles to utilize fuel more effectively resulting in a greater level of exercising. (moveit4.org)

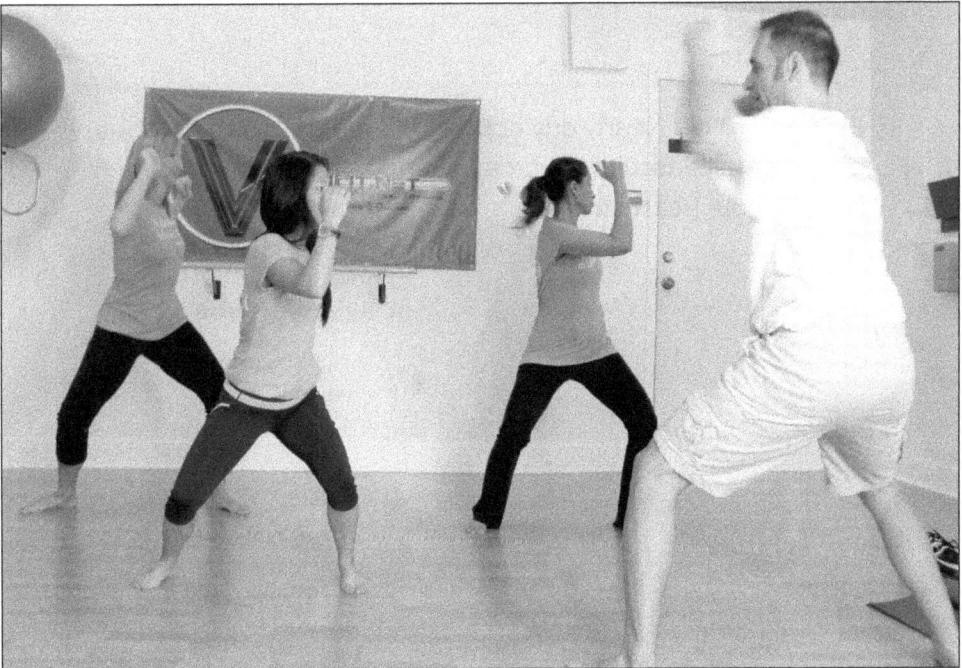

Torso Twists for Warmup

CARDIO ACTIVITIES

Arc Trainer

Elliptical trainer

Group Exercise class

Indoor cycling (Spinning®)

Rower

Stationary bike/outdoor bike

Stepmill/Stepper

Swimming/Aquatics

Treadmill

Walking/Jogging

FITNESS TIP: Nearly any action or combinations of actions can be cardiovascular. Be creative and safe to have fun keeping your heart strong.

CARDIO BASICS

Adapt your cardiovascular routine to your goals and change as plateaus occur

Exercise in your target heart rate range, not that medication, heart conditions, athleticism, etc. may alter your range

Experiment with various programs and settings available on each machine

If seeking fat loss, work up to 30 or more minutes per cardiovascular session

Participate in various group exercise programs

Stretch after each cardiovascular session

Use intervals to keep the body guessing

Vary cardiovascular exercise: use at least three different pieces of equipment per week

Vary your intensity, duration, and frequency

Wear appropriate footwear

CARDIO BENEFITS

Changes body composition

Decreases body fat

Improves cardiovascular health

Improves circulation

Improves recovery

Increases endurance

Increases energy

Lowers blood pressure

Reduces risk of heart disease

Strengthens heart

FITNESS TIP: Find the target heart rate for cardio that gives you the best results and the best feeling.

CARDIO HAZARDS

Improper biomechanical alignment (consult personal trainer for proper alignment)

Improper footwear

Injuries from repetitive exercise (lack of variety)

Loose form on rower, using lower back rather than upper back

Losing focus, especially when on the treadmill

Missing step on stepmill

Poor running form

Running heavy, too much impact on feet

Running with weights

Veering from center of treadmill

FITNESS TIP: Understanding and executing how our core works in all movements made is a fundamental process of health.

BODY WEIGHT PLYOMETRIC BASIC

Butt kickers

Forward hops

Hi knees

Hops

Side hops

Squat jumps

Stair hops

Stair jogging

Stationary jogging

Note: Perform 2 rounds consisting of 45 seconds with break between rounds. Vary duration and break time.

BODY WEIGHT PLYOMETRIC INTERMEDIATE

Band archer row

Box hops

Clap pushup

Floor tricep dip hops

Forward hops

Hop and chop

Jump lunge

Lateral box leaps

Lateral leaps

Mason twist

Note: Perform 3 rounds consisting of 60 seconds with break between rounds. Vary duration and break time.

BODY WEIGHT PLYOMETRIC ADVANCED

Bar or broomstick twist

Box leaps

Clap close grip pushup

Dumbbell bent over pass row, one arm row and pass to other hand while rowing, alternating hands

Forward leaps

High/low plank

Lateral box hops

Lateral hops

Stability ball pop pushups

Vertical leap

Note: Between each exercise do 10 situps, 10 pushups, 10 pull ups or rows and ten burpees.

BODY WEIGHT CARDIO BASIC

Chinese drum

Jogging

Runners

Slow jog in place

Squats

Stair jogging

Toe Touch

Walking

Walking stairs

Note: Perform 2 rounds, the first for 30 seconds and the second for 45 seconds

BODY WEIGHT CARDIO INTERMEDIATE

1. Jumping jacks

2. Tricep dip

3. Side jump lunge

4. Pushup

5. Low jacks

6. Superman

7. V half burpees

8. One leg deadlift

9. Mountain climbers

10. Supine leg lift

11. Burpees

12. Bicycles

Note: Perform 2 rounds, the first for 30 seconds and the second for 60 seconds.

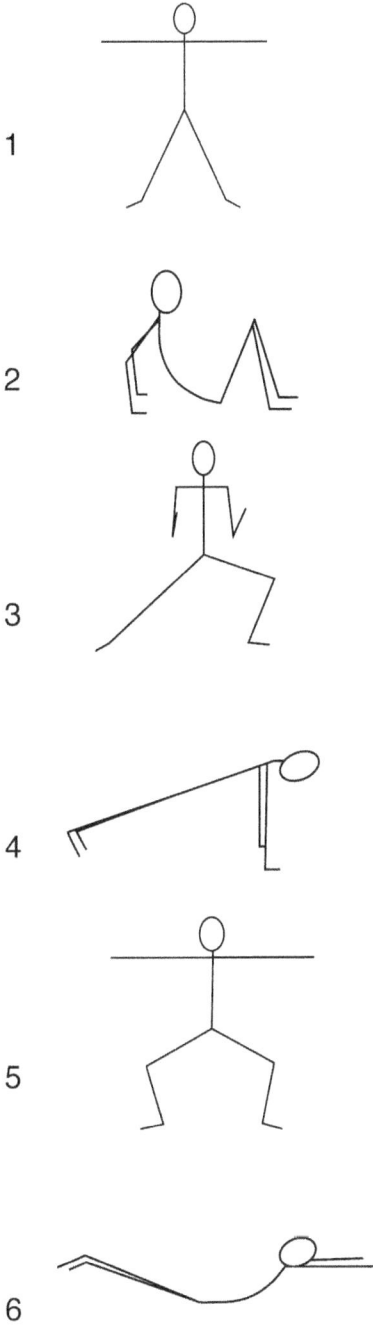

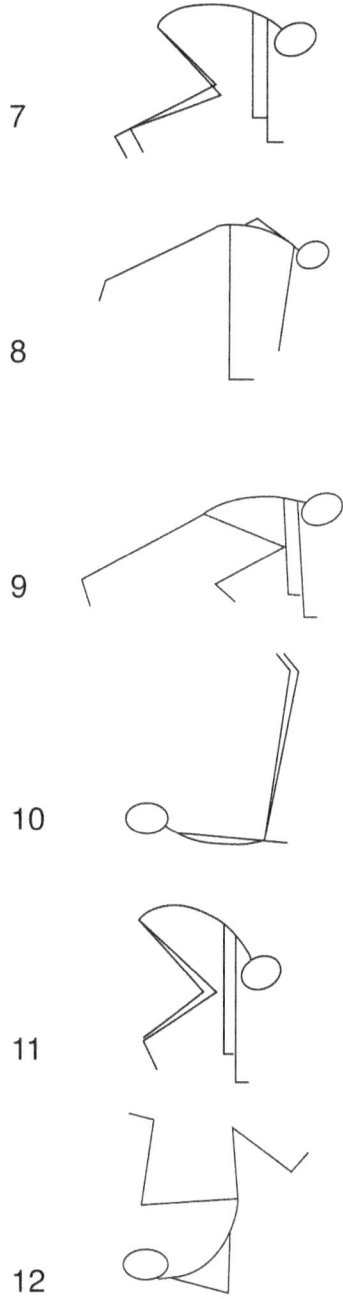

BODY WEIGHT CARDIO ADVANCED

1. Runners

2. Get ups

3. Crisscross

4. Burpees

5. Teaser/paulina

6. Pushup knee to elbow

7. Half burpees

8. Jump squat

9. Incline plane/situp toe touch

10. Jump lunge

11. Ninja jumps

12. High/low plank

13. Superdog

14. Swimmers

15. Scorpion

16. Burpees with pushup

Note: Perform 3 rounds consisting of 30 seconds, 60 seconds, and 90 seconds.

1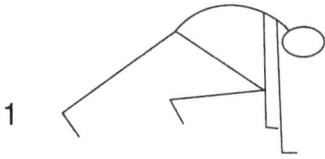

5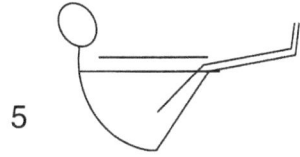

2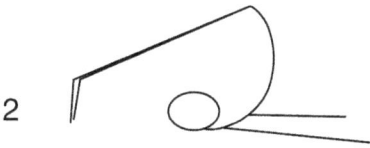

6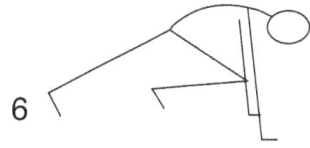

3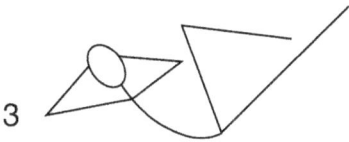

7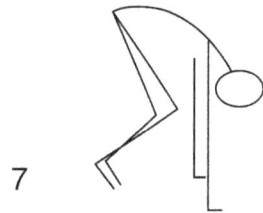

4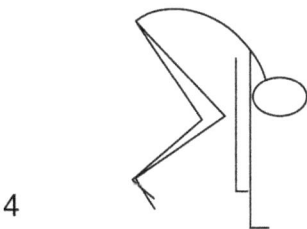

8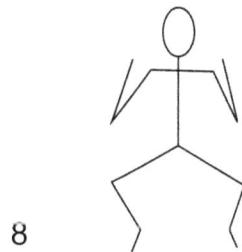

9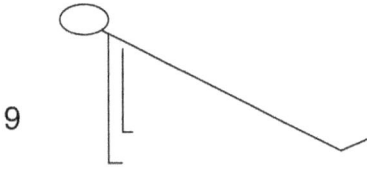

13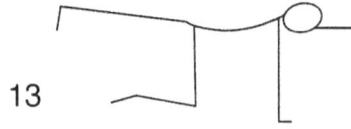

10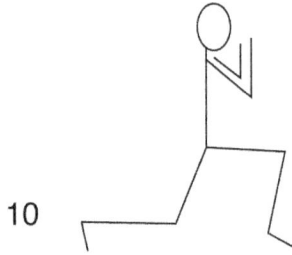

14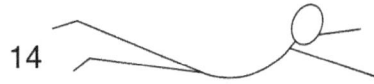

11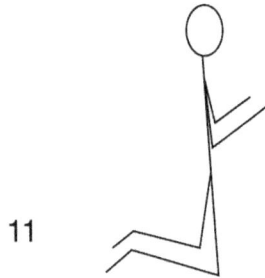

15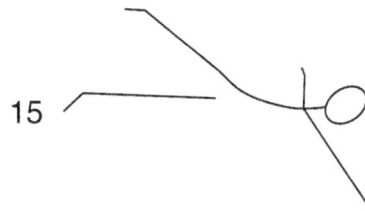

12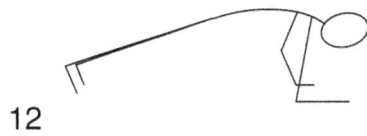

16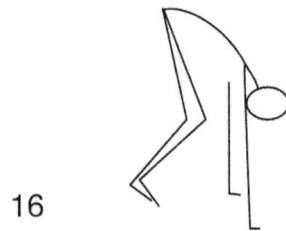

BODY WEIGHT CONDITIONING

1. Squat

2. Floor tricep dip

3. Crunch

4. One leg balance, eyes closed

5. Calf raise

6. Down dog pushup

7. Side lying crunch

8. Balance on toes, eyes closed

9. Back lunge

10. Supine lat pullover

11. Superman/bow pose

12. Heel-toe line walk, eyes closed

13. Asymmetric grip pushup

14. Bridge lift

15. Paulina

16. Contralateral pushup balance

Note: Perform 3 rounds consisting of 60 seconds with break between rounds.

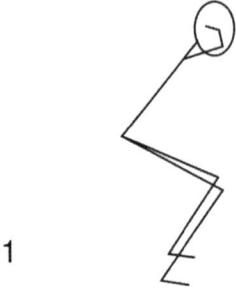

1

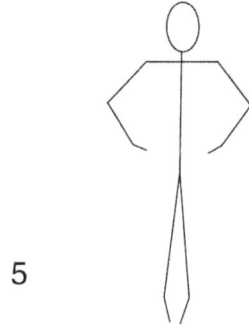

5

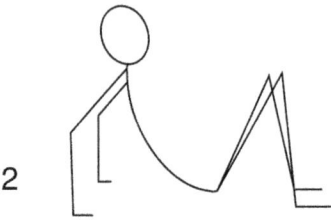

2

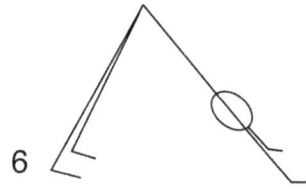

6

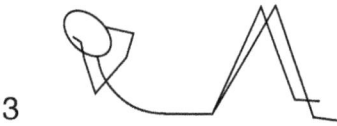

3

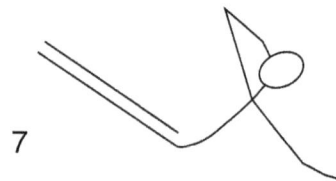

7

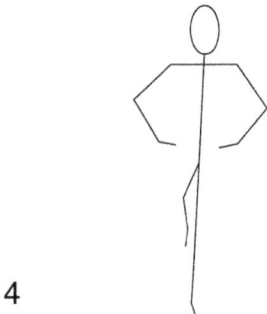

4

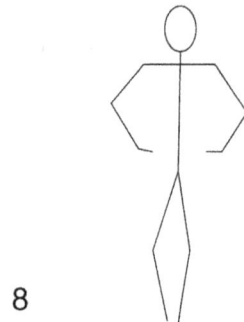

8

9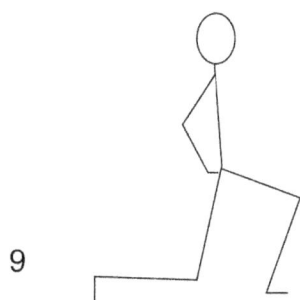

13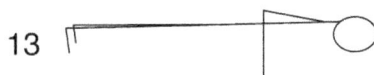

10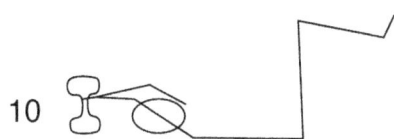

14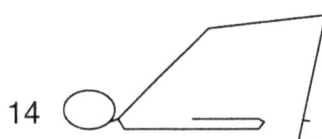

11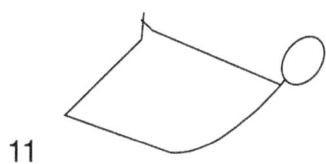

15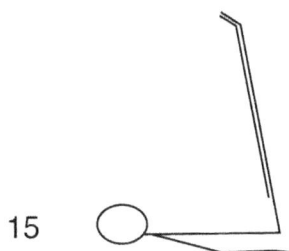

12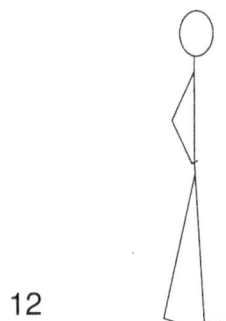

16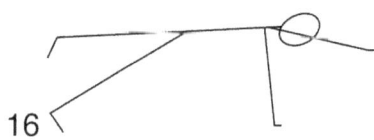

BOSU® BALL CARDIO

1. Squat hop laterally over ball

2. Jumping jacks on and off ball

3. Jump lunge, lead leg on ball

4. V half burpees, holding inverted ball

5. Superman, ball under torso

6. Burpees, holding inverted ball

7. Pop pushup, holding inverted ball

8. Mountain climber, holding inverted ball

9. High knees on ball

10. Butt kickers on ball

Note: Perform 3 rounds consisting of 30 seconds, 60 seconds, and 90 seconds.

1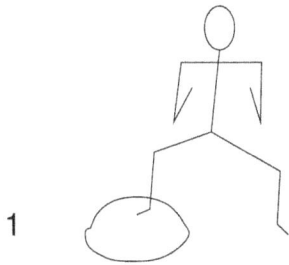

6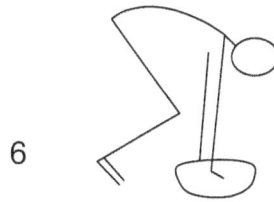

2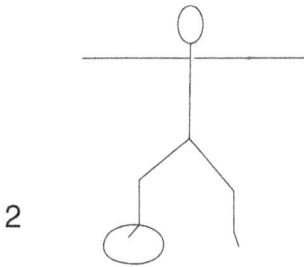

7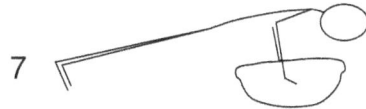

3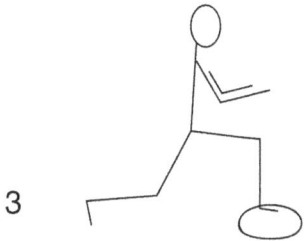

8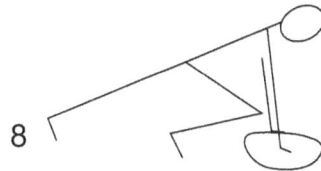

4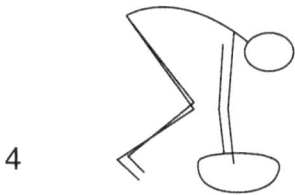

9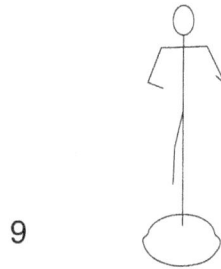

5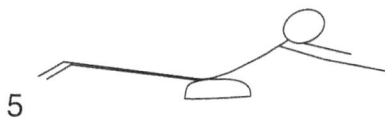

10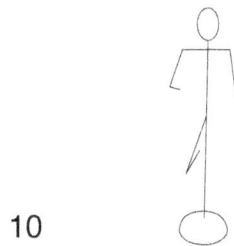

BOSU® BALL CONDITIONING

Low side plank hip lift, forearm on ball

Get ups, holding inverted ball

Burpees with pushup, holding inverted ball

Wide leg half burpees, holding inverted ball

Ninja jumps on ball

Skiers on ball

Deep squat on ball

Jump squat with high knee tuck on ball

Jump lunge, lead leg on ball

Note: Perform 3 rounds consisting of 60 seconds with break between rounds.

FITNESS TIP: Boxing training incorporates many aspects of total fitness.

BOSU® BALL PLYOMETRIC

Jump squats, on ball

Alternating twist crunches, low back on ball

Pop pushup, holding ball upside down

Alternating jump lunges, one foot on ball

Medicine ball ab crunches, low back on ball

One arm row, other hand on ball

Straight leg ball hops, on ball

Alternating arm-leg lift, all fours on ball

Hi-Lo plank, forearms on ball

Mason twist, seated on ball

Superman, lying on ball

Note: Perform 3 rounds consisting of 60 seconds with break between rounds. Vary duration and break time.

CALISTHENIC PLYOMETRIC

1. Pushup

2. Squat

3. Pull up or chin up

4. Jump squat

5. Squat and thrust

6. Situp

7. Supine leg raise

8. Handstand

9. Forward lunge

10. Back lunge

Note: Perform 3 rounds consisting of 60 seconds with break between

1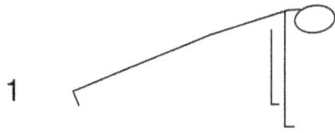

6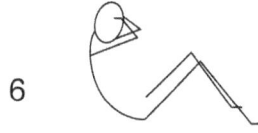

2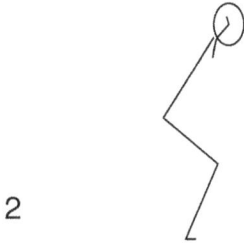

7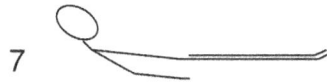

3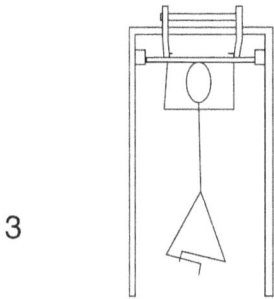

8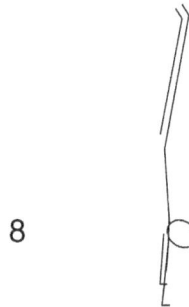

4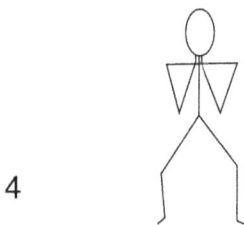

9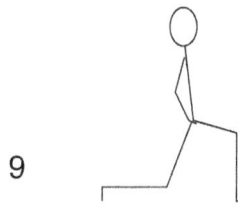

5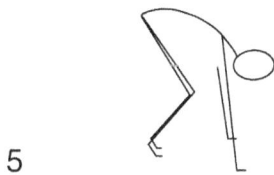

10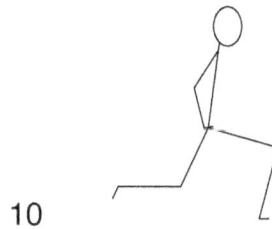

CARDIO CORE WORKOUT 1

Supine one leg hip lift/crunch

Supine wide leg lift/paulina

Mountain climbers

Wide leg burpees/pushup

Ninja jumps/half burpees

Side lateral hop with two hand touch

Squat with lateral kick

Jump squat with two hand touch

One leg deadlift

Note: Repeat 2–4 times.

CARDIO CORE WORKOUT 2

Reverse tabletop contralateral lift

Get ups

Alternating one leg pushup

Burpees

Half wide leg burpees/pushup

Side lateral hop, elbows touch floor

Pulse squat

Jump squat with kick

Circle squat

Note: Repeat 2–4 times.

CARDIO CORE WORKOUT 3

V situp/paulina

Side lying V crunch

Santana pushup

Runners

Wide leg burpees

Half burpees/pushup

Ice skaters

Jump squat

Standing kick over chair

Note: Repeat 2–4 times.

CARDIO CORE WORKOUT 4

Situp/knee in

Paulina

Pushup with alternating lateral leg lift

Half burpees

Ninja jumps/tucks

Hop skaters

Deep squat/back extension

180 Jump squat

Pulse lunge

Note: Repeat 2–4 times.

CARDIO CORE WORKOUT 5

Jump squat

Up dog/Down dog

Clap pushup

Deep squat

Paulina/Plow

Half burpees

Walking lunge

Situp/Crunch

Burpees

Note: 3 rounds: first round 30 seconds each exercise, second round 45 seconds, third round 60 seconds. If necessary, add fourth round 90 seconds each.

CARDIO CORE WORKOUT 6

Jump lunge

Hi plank/Low plank

Santana pushup

Hi knees

Hi cable ab crunch

Crab walks

Alternating one-leg hop squat

Mason twist with dumbbell

Jump burpee with pushup

Sprints

Note: 3 rounds: first round 30 seconds each exercise, second round 45 seconds, third round 60 seconds. If necessary, add fourth round 90 seconds each.

CARDIO CORE WORKOUT 7

Jog in place

Medicine ball situp

Pullups

Butt kickers

Speed situp

Hi plank walk (pushup walk)

Jumping jacks

Teaser

Runners

Sprints

Note: 3 rounds: first round 30 seconds each exercise, second round 45 seconds, third round 60 seconds. If necessary, add fourth round 90 seconds each.

CARDIO CORE WORKOUT 8

Treadmill, highest incline

Ab rollout

Squat/Dumbbell shoulder press

Groucho squat walk

Superman swimmer

Bent-over alternating dumbbell speed rows

Inch worm

Superman/Up bow

Mountain climber

Sprints

Note: 3 rounds: first round 30 seconds each exercise, second round 45 seconds, third round 60 seconds. If necessary, add fourth round 90 seconds each.

CARDIO "YOGA"

Sun Salutation A

Sun Salutation B

Sun Salutation B with high lunge

Sun Salutation B with warrior II

Sun Salutation B with warrior III

Sun Salutation B

Sun Salutation A

Note: This is not yoga, there are no poses. Participants flow from position to position with only a 1–2 second pause at each traditional pose. We use the transition movements from yoga from pose to pose to form a cardio activity.

MARATHON BASICS

Clear mind

Cross training

Don't over think

Establish pace

Gu® gel, energy replacement

Heart rate monitor/pacer

One long run per week

Positive attitude

Proper footwear

Weekly massage

PLYOMETRIC CORE

1. Medicine ball situp

2. Medicine ball situp throwing ball to partner

3. Medicine ball overhead front throw to partner

4. Medicine ball overhead backward throw to partner

5. Medicine ball speed twist situp

6. Spiderman crawl on floor

7. Drop pushup

8. Drop pushup/jog interval

9. Jump squat and thrust

10. Seated medicine ball twist and throw

Note: Perform 3 rounds consisting of 60 seconds with break between rounds. Vary duration and break time. Or perform 3 rounds consisting of 15–25 reps with break between rounds. Vary reps and break time. Medicine ball can be rebounded to a wall if available.

1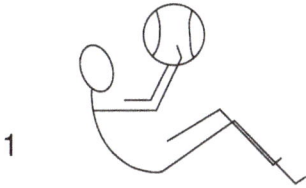

6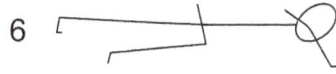

2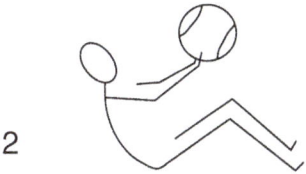

7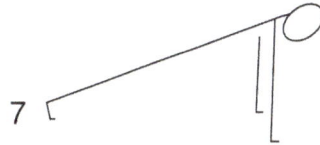

3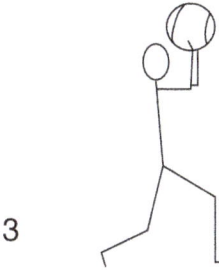

8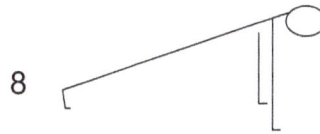

4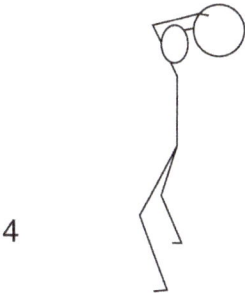

9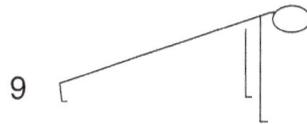

5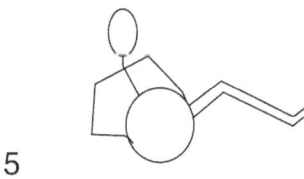

10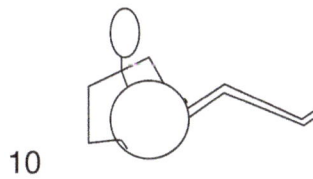

PLYOMETRIC LOWER BODY

1. Jump squat

2. Lateral hop

3. Split jack

4. Standing triple jump

5. Standing long jump

6. Box jump or depth jump

7. Standing calf jump

8. Jumping jacks

9. Jumping rope

10. Back jump

Note: Perform 3 rounds consisting of 60 seconds with break between rounds. Vary duration and break time.

1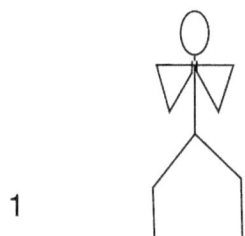

2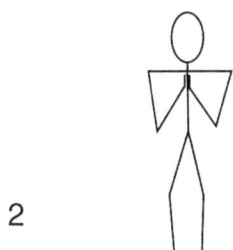

3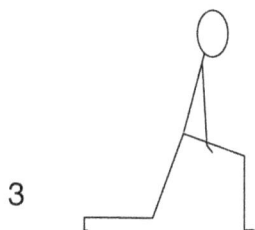

4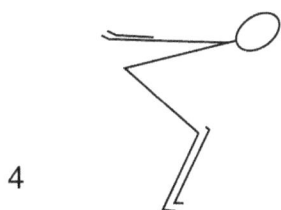

5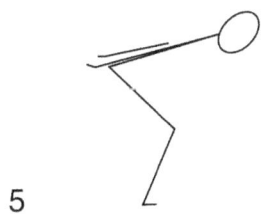

6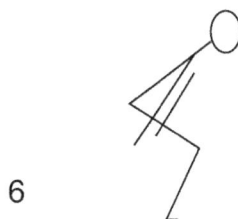

7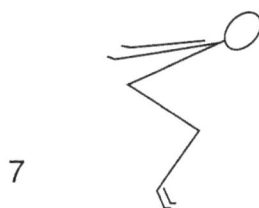

8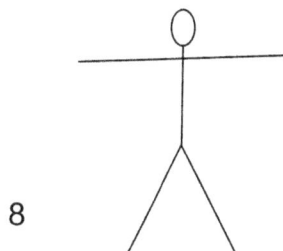

9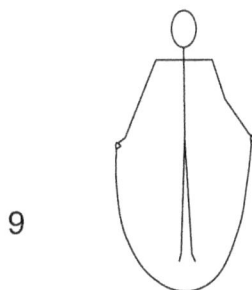

10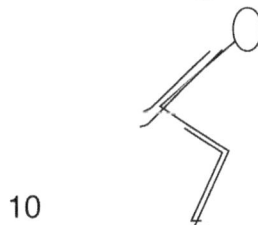

PLYOMETRIC UPPER BODY

Clap pushup

Dumbbell arm swing

Medicine ball overhead backward throw

Drop pushup

Jump negative chin

Step plyometric pushup

Walking on hands

Medicine ball overhead front throw

Explosive tricep dip

Jump squat and overhead dumbbell push

Note: Perform 3 rounds consisting of 60 seconds with break between rounds. Vary duration and break time.

RUNNING BASICS

Run no more than 3 times per week

Purchase appropriate footwear

Stay mentally and physically relaxed

Move naturally/keep consistent stride

Keep form neutral and relaxed

Run within your limits/biomechanics

Avoid ball first or heel first impact

Keep a rhythm and pump arms

Stay alert

Wear a heart monitor

Note: Tai Chi can also be a great warmup for running.

STAIRWELL TRAINING

Stair walking

Stair jogging

Stair sprinting

Step laterals, walking sideways on stairwell

Step laterals, doubles, every other step

Stair springing doubles, every other step

Stair springing triples, every third step

Weighted stair running

Stair intervals, performing body weight exercises at top of stairs with stair running between sets

Calf raise intervals, performing a set of calf raises at bottom of steps, run up stairs and back down to next to bottom step, repeat until at top of stair

Note: It is not recommended to run down stairs

STABILITY BALL PLYOMETRIC BASIC

Squat, ball between low back and wall

Standing, balance on stability ball with support

Bridge on stability ball

Low plank, forearms on stability ball

Crunch, feet on floor, low back on stability ball

Bent over single arm row, one hand on stability ball

Wall pushup, hands on stability ball

Tricep dip, hands on stability ball

Note: Perform 3 rounds consisting of 30 seconds with break between rounds. Vary duration and break time.

STABILITY BALL PLYOMETRIC INTERMEDIATE

1. Squat, ball between low back and wall

2. Chair, seated balance on stability ball

3. Standing, balance on stability ball with support

4. Alternating single leg lift hip lift, feet on stability ball

5. Low plank rollout, forearms on stability ball

6. Crunch, alternate leg lift, feet on floor, low back on stability ball

7. Bent over single arm row, one hand on stability ball, contralateral leg lifted

8. Wall pushup, hands on stability ball

9. Tuck pushup, knees on stability ball, hands on floor, head tucked, for deltoids

10. Tricep dip, hands on stability ball

Note: Perform 3 rounds consisting of 30 seconds with break between rounds. Vary duration and break time.

1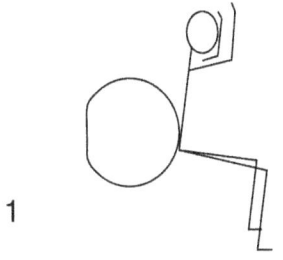

6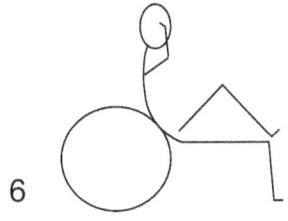

2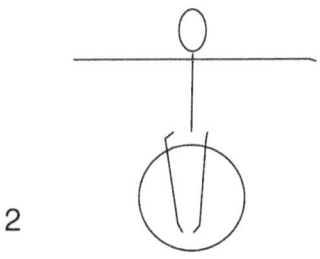

7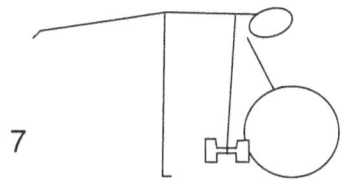

3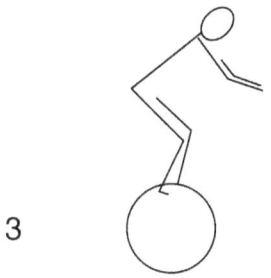

8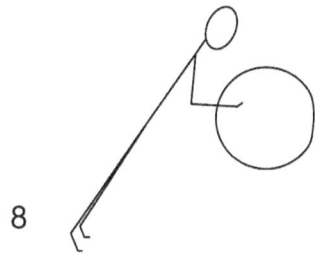

4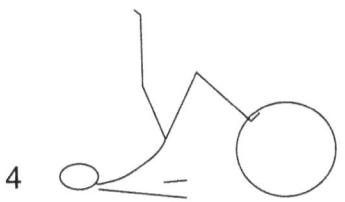

9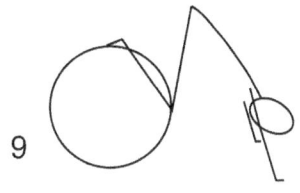

5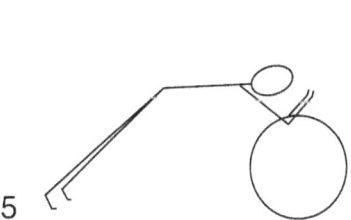

10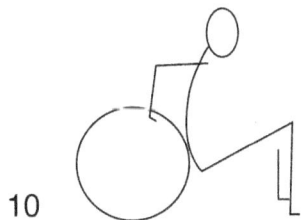

STABILITY BALL PLYOMETRIC ADVANCED

1. Squat, standing on stability ball with support

2. Bulgarian squat, one leg on stability ball

3. Kneeling balance, shins on stability ball

4. Alternating straight leg lift, heels on stability ball

5. Crunch ball transfer, transfer stability ball from hands to ankles while crunching

6. Side lying one leg lift, feet on stability ball

7. Pull up, feet on stability ball

8. Clock pushup, feet on stability ball

9. Standing one arm pushup, hand on stability ball on wall

10. Close grip pushup, hands on stability ball

Note: Between each exercise do 10 crunch ball transfers, 10 pushups hands on stability ball, 10 pull ups or rows, 10 burpees holding stability ball

1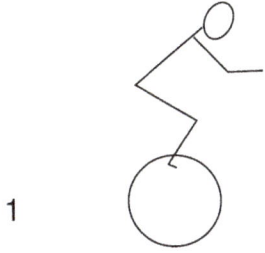

6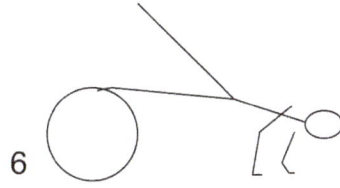

2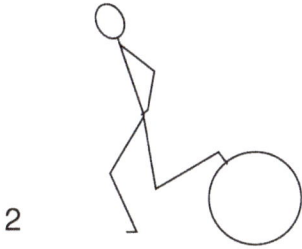

7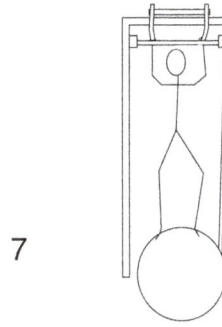

3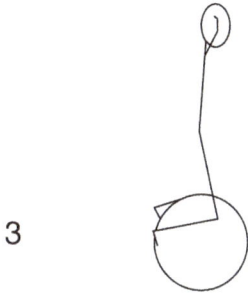

8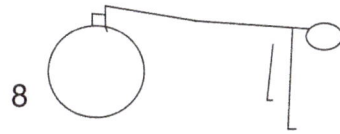

4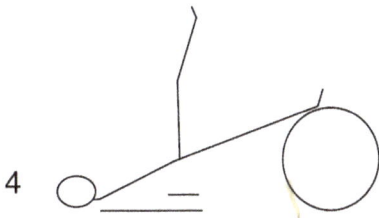

9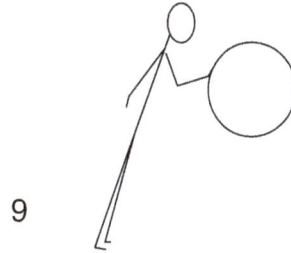

5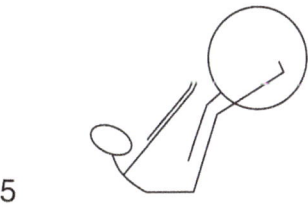

10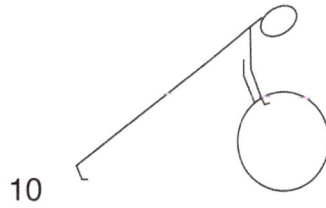

STEP CONDITIONING

1. Step ups

2. Situp, legs on step

3. Pushup, feet on step

4. Lateral step ups

5. Crunch, legs on step

6. Tricep dip, hands on step

7. Step up splits

8. Pull ups or vertical row

9. Step hop ups

10. Low plank, feet on step

11. Step hop overs

12. Low side plank, feet on step

Note: Equipment is required for Pull ups or Rows. Substitute Superman swimmers if no equipment available.

1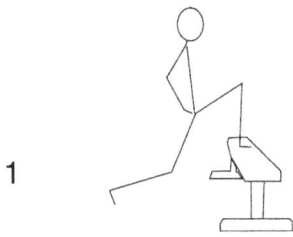

7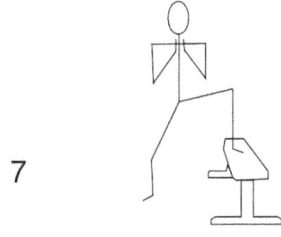

2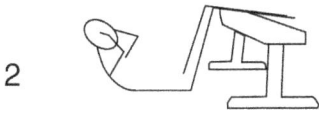

8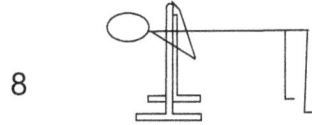

3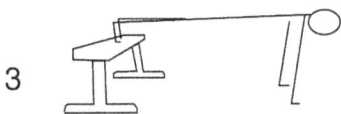

9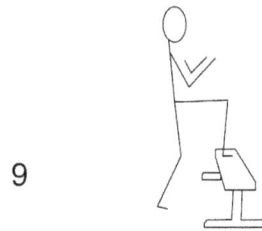

4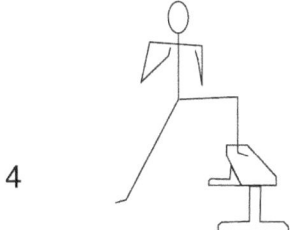

10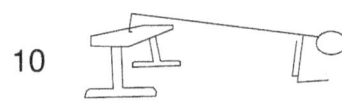

5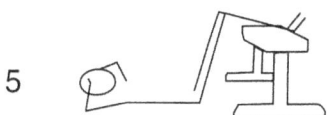

11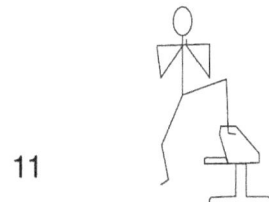

6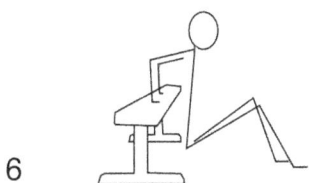

12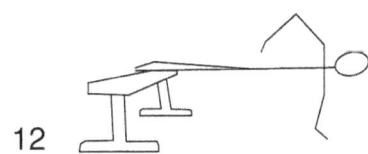

TOP CARDIOVASCULAR CALORIE BURNERS

Bicycling

Cross-country skiing

Elliptical machines

Hiking

Indoor cycling (Spinning®)

Jogging Stairs

Rowing machines

Running

Step aerobics

Swimming

Reference: Top 10 Cardio exercises, exercise.about.com, ©2005

TREADMILL TRAINING

Lunging

Laterals

Climbs on highest incline

Sprints

Walking intervals

Sprinting intervals

Lunge with hip extension

Laterals with hip abduction

Walking backward

Jogging backward

Walking backward

Jogging with dumbbells

Walking backward

Jogging using dumbbells with upper body movement

Note: Caution, perform exercises if confident of abilities. Perform 2 rounds consisting of 60 seconds with break between rounds

WARMING UP BASICS

Gradually increase intensity

If you rest more than 5 minutes, warm up again
before continuing

Keep room and body temp moderate

Start slow

Stretch

Use as many joints as possible

Use cardiovascular equipment

Use full range of motion

Use jumping jacks or jump rope

Use self-myofascial release

FITNESS TIP: Buy organic foods and products from
independently companies.

WARMING UP EXERCISES

Alternate toe touch

Burpees

Chinese drum

Jog in place

Jump rope

Jump squat

Jumping jacks

Medicine ball circuit

Proper ballistic movements

Shuttle running

Split jacks

Stair running

Note: This is a great way to warm up before any workout. Pick 5 or 6 and perform for one minute each and then bring on the fitness!

WARMING UP WITHOUT EQUIPMENT

Alternate toe touches

Burpees

Jog in place

Jump rope

Jump squat

Jumping jacks/split jacks

Medicine ball circuit

Proper ballistic movements

Shuttle running

Stair running

FITNESS TIP: Any repetitive functional movement that raises the heart rate can produce an effective warmup. Be creative.

WALKING BASICS

Bend elbows

Breathe fully and continually

Don't lean forward or back

Hold neutral spine, keep core engaged

Let foot hit the ground properly and gently

Move arms

Purchase appropriate sneakers for any foot
or ankle condition

Relax shoulders

Stay alert

Stay mentally and physically relaxed

FITNESS TIP: Enjoy the mental and spiritual aspect of walking as well. Yoga can be a wonderful cool down activity after a walk.

X-CYCLING

Bike, warm up

Jumping jacks, one minute

Bike, sprints

Pull up or vertical row, one minute

Bike, climbs

Pushup, one minute

Bike, jumps

Situp or crunch, one minute

Bike, sprints

Squat, one minute

Bike, climbs

Deadlift with dumbbells, one minute

(continued on next page)

X-CYCLING (Cont.)

Bike, jumps

Lunge, one minute

Bike, sprints

Tricep dip, one minute

Bike, climbs

Dumbbell bicep curl, one minute

Bike, jumps

Burpees

Bike, cool down

Stretch

Note: X-Cycling is a cross training class with an indoor cycling bike. Participants train one song on the bike, the next off the bike. Each bike portion is about four minutes long, Each floor work is about one to two minutes long. This is approximately an hour class.

YOGA WARMUPS

Sun Salutations A

Sun Salutations B

Moon Salutations 1

Moon Salutations 2

Moon Salutations 3

Cardio "yoga" (see page 30)

Note: See Yoga Sun Salutations A or B or Yoga Moon Salutations 1, 2 or 3 in the Pilates & Yoga Chapter for details of using yoga as a warmup.

FITNESS TIP: The key to warming up safely in two-fold, proper form and proper breathwork.

CHAPTER 2

Muscular & Resistance Workouts

RESISTANCE TRAINING is a form of strength training in which each effort is performed against a specific opposing force generated by resistance (i.e. resistance to being pushed, squeezed, stretched or bent). Exercises are isotonic if a body part is moving against the force. Exercises are isometric if a body part is holding still against the force. Resistance exercise is used to develop the strength and size of skeletal muscles. Properly performed, resistance training can provide significant functional benefits and improvement in overall health and well-being. (en.wikipedia.org)

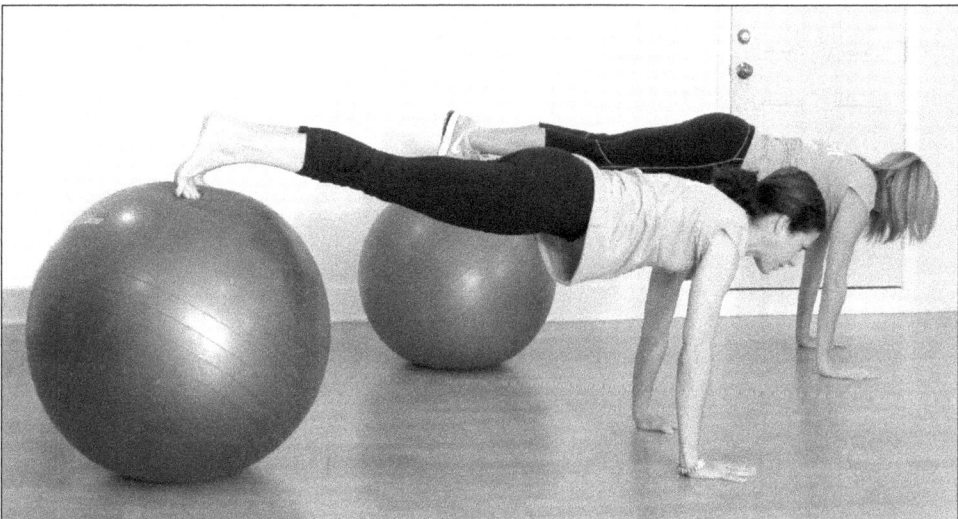

Stability ball pushups

AB WHEEL WORKOUT

Kneeling rollout

Kneeling rollout, arcing to side

Kneeling rollout, alternate arcing to side

Standing drop to knees rollout

Standing rollout into wall, wall acts as safety stop

One knee rollout

Alternating one knee rollout

Kneeling rollout on Bosu® ball

Note: Perform 3 rounds consisting of 30 seconds with break between rounds. Vary duration and break time.

ADDING VARIETY TO WORKOUTS

Combine supersets with pyramid or drop sets.

Cut your weight in half and do high reps, 30 or more

Do 100's: Select an exercise with your normal weight and perform until you do 100 reps, breaking as needed for 5–10 seconds

Perform 30 minutes of weight resistance with no breaks, must have weights prepared or machine pre-loaded

Perform a cardiovascular activity for 20 seconds between each resistance exercise (eg, burpees, jumping jacks, etc.)

Perform exercise on one-leg with eyes closed, consider safety concerns

Perform exercises while balancing on a stability ball, assure ball is burst proof

Perform reps in slo-mo, 5 seconds per rep or longer

Reduce you rest period by 50–75%

Use asymmetry dumbbell loads, heavier weight in weaker hand

BAND WORKOUT

1. Band squat

2. Band crunch

3. Band row

4. Band lunge

5. Band ab twist

6. Band chest press

7. Band calf raise

8. Superman or Birddog

9. Band tricep extension

10. Band bicep curl

Note: Perform 3 rounds consisting of 30 seconds with break between rounds. Vary duration and break time.

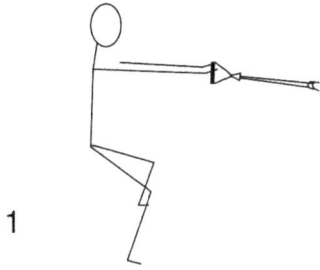

1

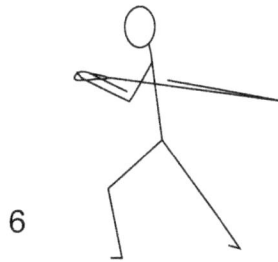

6

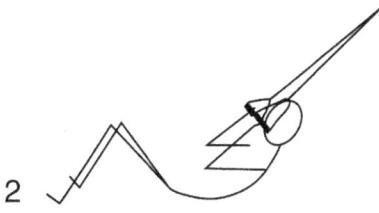

2

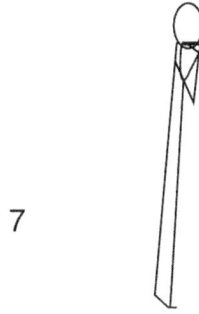

7

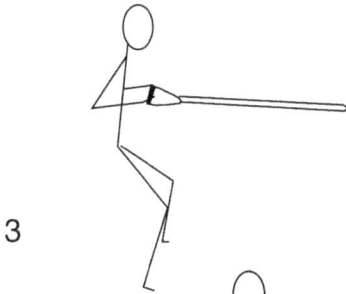

3

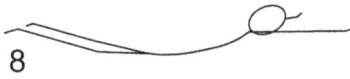

8

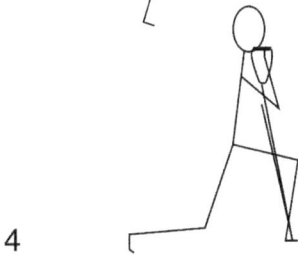

4

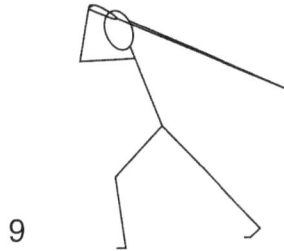

9

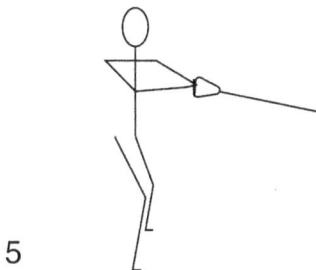

5

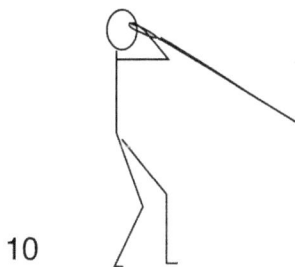

10

ABDOMINAL EXERCISES

Bench reverse crunch

Crunch

Kneeling cable crunch

Machine crunch

Medicine ball plyometric situp

Reverse crunch

Rollout with wheel or stability ball

Situp

V situp

Wood chop

Note: Perform 3 rounds consisting of 15–25 reps with break between rounds. Vary reps and break time. Perform with fullest range of motion available. Avoid hyperextending lumbars.

BODY WEIGHT CORE WORKOUT BASIC

Situp

Seated knee in

Seated side bend

Superman

Supine leg raise

Prone leg raise

Supine crunch

Boat pose

Note: Perform 3 rounds consisting of 30 seconds with break between rounds. Vary duration and break time. Or perform 3 rounds consisting of 15–25 reps with break between rounds. Vary reps and break time.

BODY WEIGHT CORE WORKOUT INTERMEDIATE

1. Situp toe touch

2. Seated knee in

3. Lying side crunch

4. Superman

5. Teaser

6. Supine leg raise

7. Supine cork screw

8. Prone leg raise

9. Supine pulse crunch

10. Seated mason twist

Note: Perform 3 rounds consisting of 30 seconds with break between rounds. Vary duration and break time. Or perform 3 rounds consisting of 15–25 reps with break between rounds. Vary reps and break time.

1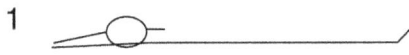

6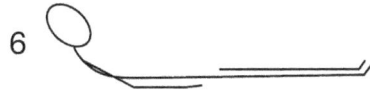

2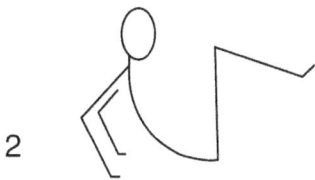

7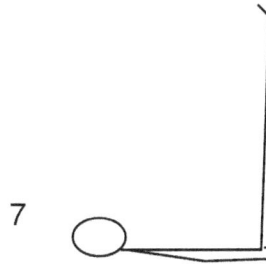

3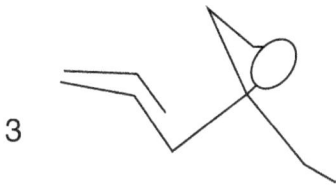

8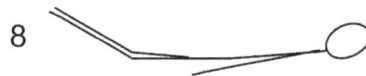

4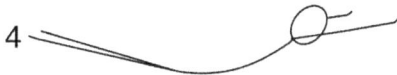

9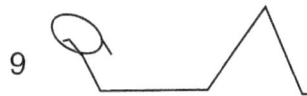

5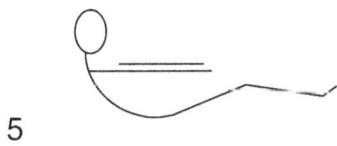

10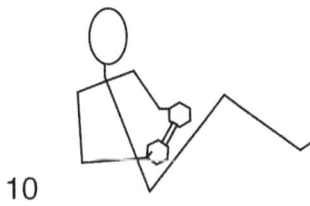

BODY WEIGHT CORE WORKOUT ADVANCED

1. Jump lunge, two hand touch

2. Ice skaters

3. Wood chop

4. Lateral hop, two hand touch

5. One leg deadlift

6. Standing twist

7. Jump squat, two hand touch

8. Tae Bo® goddess twist

9. Up dog/down dog

10. Reverse tabletop contralateral lift

11. Mountain climbers

12. High/low plank

13. Corkscrew

14. Situp/knee in

15. Superman

16. Savasana/plow

Note: Between each exercise do 10 situps, 10 pushups and 10 pull ups or rows

1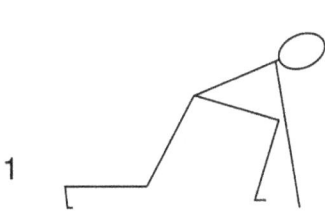

5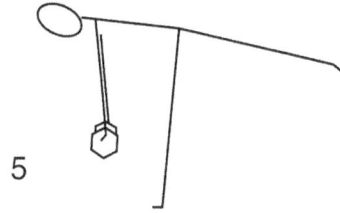

2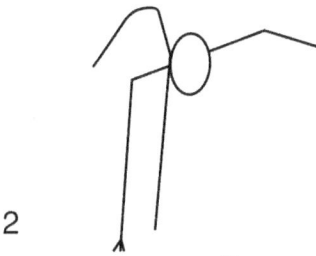

6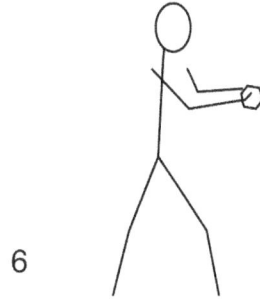

3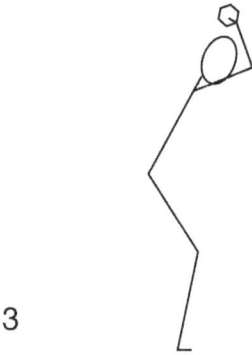

7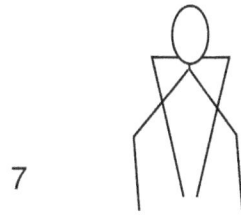

4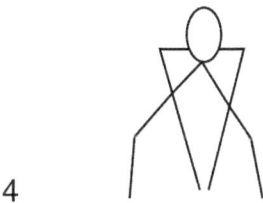

8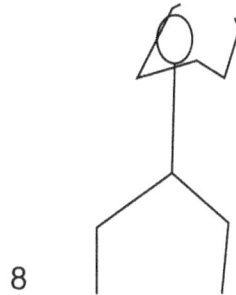

9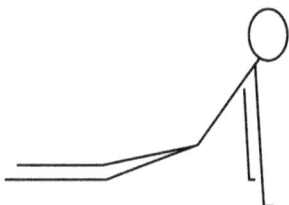

13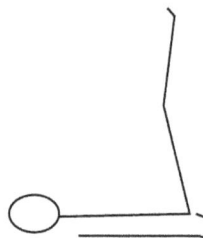

10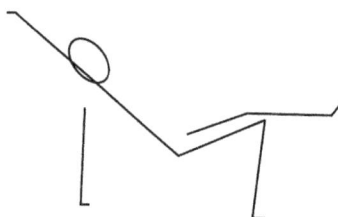

14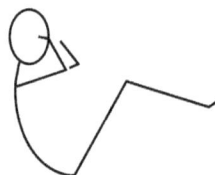

11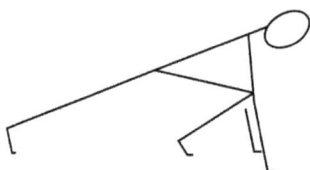

15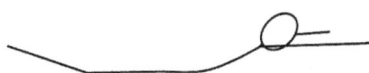

12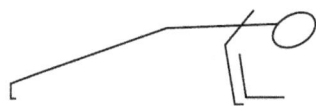

16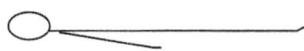

BICEP EXERCISES

Barbell bicep curl

Dumbbell bicep curl

Preacher bicep curl

Low cable bicep curl

Concentration bicep curl

High cable bicep curl

Negative chin

Chin up or partial chin up

Bicep dumbbell curl 21's

Note: Perform with fullest range of motion available. Avoid hyperextending elbows

BODY WEIGHT WORKOUT FULL BODY

1. Squat

2. Back Lunge

3. Birddog

4. Superman

5. Supine jackknife crunch

6. One leg calf raise

7. Recline pull up

8. Tricep dip

9. Bicep curl

10. Pushup

Note: Perform 3 rounds consisting of 30 seconds with break between rounds. Vary duration and break time.

1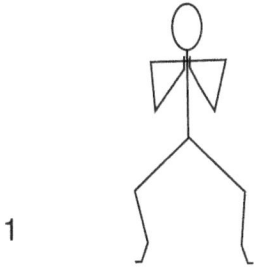

6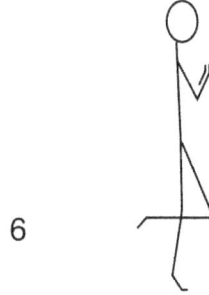

2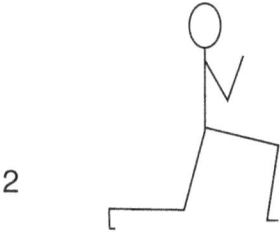

7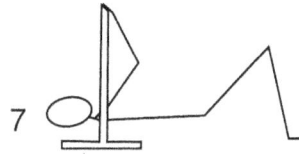

3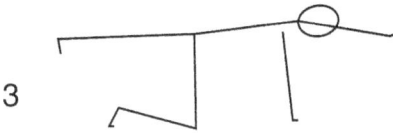

8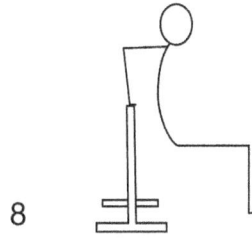

4 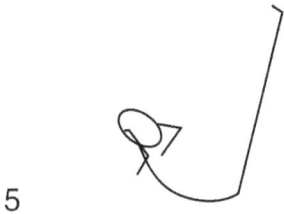 9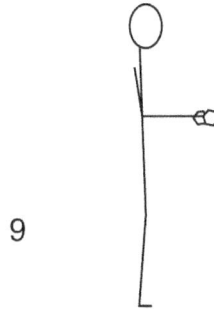

5 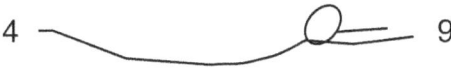 10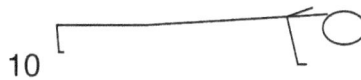

BODY WEIGHT WORKOUT UPPER BODY

1. Bridge lat pullover

2. Hip lift/wheel pose

3. Side plank arm raise

4. Side plank arm raise, switch sides

5. Superdog

6. Floor tricep dip

7. Reverse table pose

8. Curl grip pull up or standing bicep curl

9. Superman isometric, arms back

10. Down dog pushup

11. Handstand, tripod headstand or dolphin pose

12. Neutral grip pull ups or bent over row

13. Incline plane pose

14. Santana pushup

15. Chaturanga pose

Note: Perform 3 rounds consisting of 30 seconds with break between rounds. Vary duration and break time.

1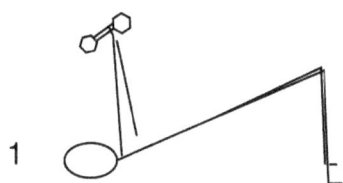

6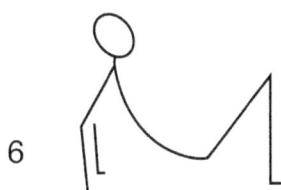

2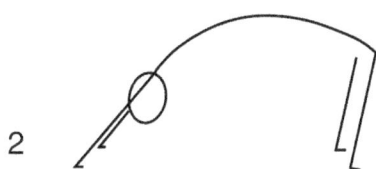

7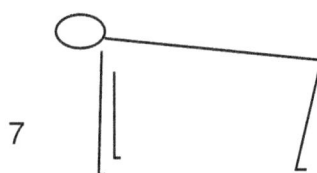

3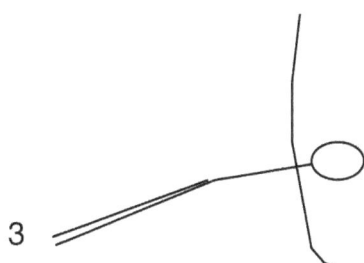

8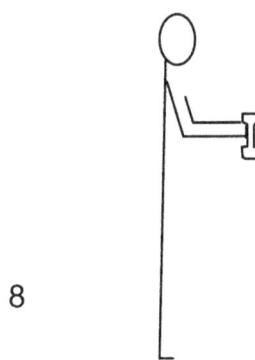

5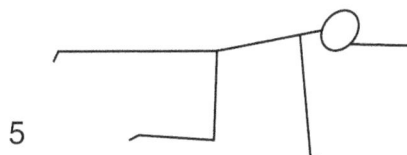

9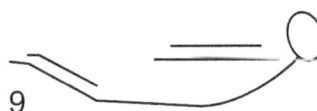

10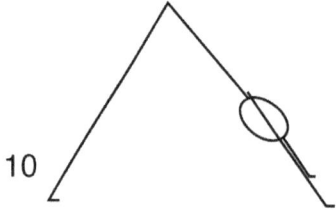

13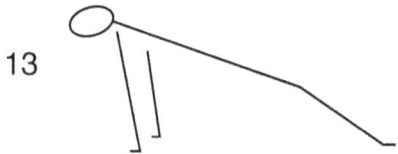

11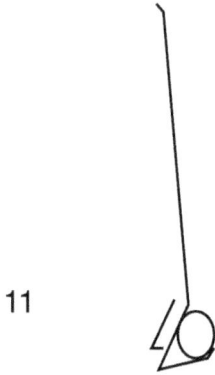

14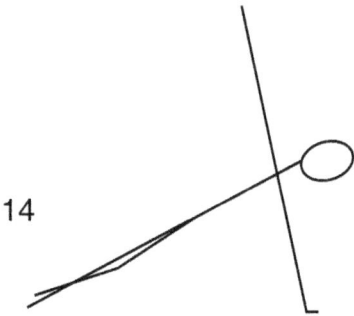

12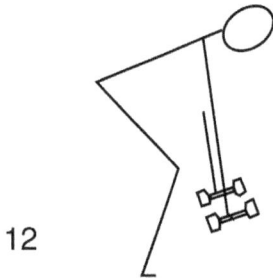

15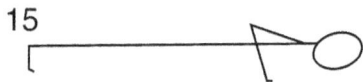

BODY WEIGHT WORKOUT LOWER BODY

Squat isometric

One leg squat

Squat

Lunge isometric

Forward lunge

Back lunge

Deadlift

One leg deadlift

Deadlift

Calf raise isometric

One leg calf raise

Calf raise

Bridge pose

One leg bridge

Hip lift

Clock lunge

Note: Perform 3 rounds consisting of 30 seconds with break between rounds. Vary duration and break time.

BOSU® BALL WORKOUT

1. Squat on ball

2. Lunge onto ball with alternating legs

3. Calf raise, toes on ball

4. Bridge, feet on ball

5. Crunch, hips on ball

6. Boat, seated on ball

7. Superman, prone on ball

8. Low side plank, forearm on ball

9. Dumbbell pullover, head/shoulders on ball

10. Pushup, hands on inverted ball

11. Dumbbell tricep overhead extension, seated on ball

12. Dumbbell bicep curl, seated on ball

Note: Perform 3 rounds consisting of 30 seconds with break between rounds. Vary duration and break time.

1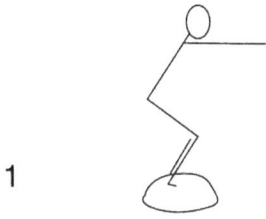

8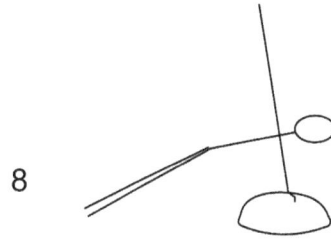

2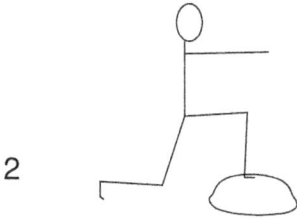

9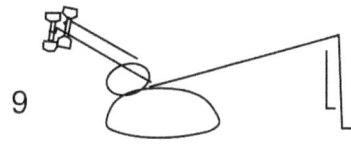

4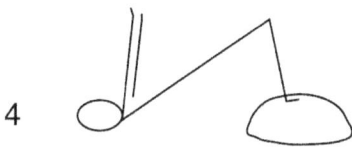

10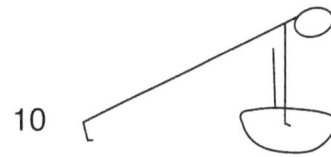

5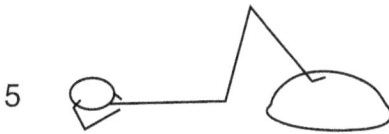

11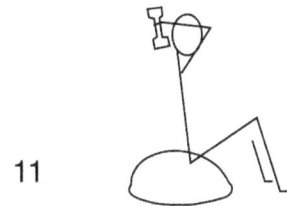

6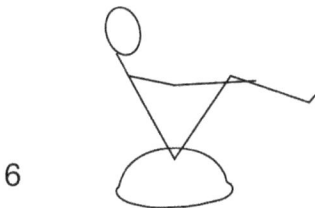

12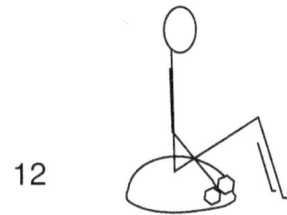

7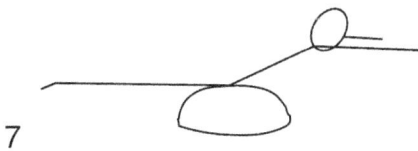

BARBELL WORKOUT

Squat

Deadlift

Upright row

Overhead press

Bent over row

Shrug

Bicep curl

Chest press

Supine overhead tricep extension chest press

Forward lunge

Note: Perform 3 rounds consisting of 30 seconds with break between rounds. Vary duration and break time.

BENEFITS OF FREE WEIGHT TRAINING

Barbells provide maximum strength

Basic

Coordination

Core balance

Dumbbells provide unilateral balance

Functional

Higher degree of focus/concentration

Inexpensive

Multi-joint

One size fits all

FITNESS TIP: Take a week off every few months to allow the body to recover. Return to exercise with new found enthusiasm.

BENEFITS OF MACHINE TRAINING

Basic

Can focus on single muscle more easily

Directions for use on machine

Easy to change weight

Energy conservation

Increase range of motion (ROM)

Isolation

Maintenance of form

Safety

Unilateral availability

FITNESS TIP: Once sound kinesiology is understood, be creative with machines to increase asymmetry and induce core use. For example, sit on a balance disk on machine while using only one limb to exercise.

BOWFLEX® WORKOUT

Seated leg press, belt required

Prone leg curl

Seated leg extension

Seated hamstring curl, belt required

Seated calf raise

Resisted ab crunch

Supine lat pulldown

Supine chest fly

Seated row

Incline chest press

Seated low back row

Standing lateral raise

Seated shoulder press

Incline tricep extension

Standing bicep curl

Note: Perform (1) first set of 15 reps, (2) second set of 10 reps, (3) third set of 8 reps, and (4) last set with 5 burpees between each set.

CORE EXERCISES

1. Corkscrew

2. Low side plank crunch, lower and lift hips

3. V situp

4. Stability ball hip lift

5. Stability ball crunch with band

6. Stability ball back extension

7. Stability ball walkout

8. Rollout with wheel or stability ball

9. Medicine ball chop

10. Medicine ball plyometric crunch, throw ball to trainer

Note: Perform 3 rounds consisting of 15–25 reps with break between rounds. Vary reps and break time.

1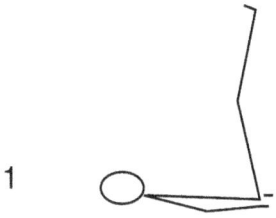

6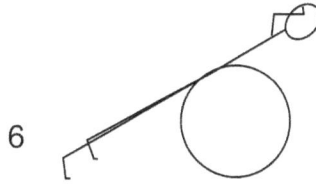

2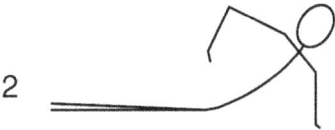

7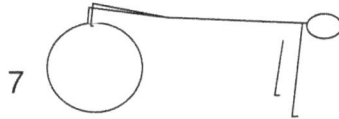

3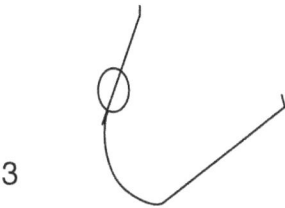

8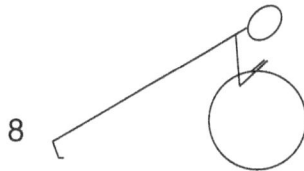

4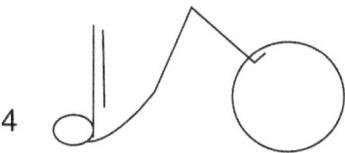

9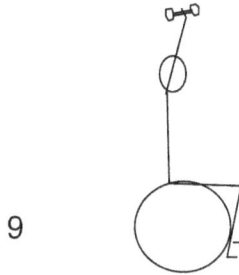

5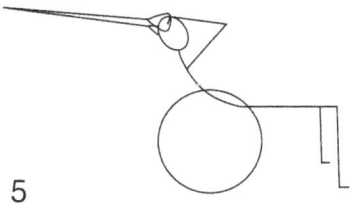

10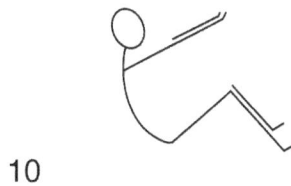

CALF EXERCISES

Donkey calf raise, partner on hips while doing bent over calf raises

Leg press calf raise

One leg jump rope

One leg jumping jacks

One leg leg press calf raise

One leg seated calf raise

One leg standing calf raise

Rotary calf machine

Seated calf raise

Standing calf raise

Note: Perform with fullest range of motion available. Occasionally perform with knees slightly bent.

CLOSED KINETIC CHAIN WORKOUT

Squats

Stationary lunges

Sissy squats

Deadlift

Pushups

Up dog/down dog

Pull ups

Tricep dip

Chin up, for biceps

Tricep dip, one leg lifted

Note: Perform 3 rounds consisting of 30 seconds with break between rounds. Vary duration and break time.

DUMBBELL WORKOUT BASIC

Dumbbell squat

Crunch

One arm row

Dumbbell lunge

Superman

Dumbbell chest press

Situp

Dumbbell tricep extension

Dumbbell side bend

Dumbbell bicep curl

Note: Perform 2 rounds consisting of 15–20 reps with break between exercises. Vary reps and break time.

DUMBBELL WORKOUT INTERMEDIATE

Dumbbell squat

Crunch

One arm row

Dumbbell deadlift

Superman

Dumbbell chest press

Dumbbell calf raise

Situp

Dumbbell tricep extension

Toe raise, for tibialis anterior

Dumbbell side bend

Dumbbell bicep curl

Dumbbell triple lunge, lunge forward, laterally,
back and repeat other leg

Note: Perform 2–3 rounds consisting of 12–25 reps with break between
rounds. Vary reps and break time. Or perform (1) first set of 15 reps,
(2) second set of 10 reps, (3) third set of 8 reps, and (4) last set with
5 burpees

DUMBBELL WORKOUT ADVANCED

1. Dumbbell tip toe squat

2. Dumbbell overhead lunge

3. Wood chop, on toes

4. One leg bent over row

5. Pullover in bridge

6. Side raise/front raise/rear fly

7. Arnold press

8. Concentration bicep curl

9. Dumbbell chest fly on stability ball, may lift one leg and hold for progression

10. One leg bent over dumbbell kickback

Note: (1) Perform each exercise with 10 crunches with dumbbells in air, 5 dumbbell Santana pushups and 10 dumbbell rows between each set. Or (2) Perform 4 rounds consisting of 12–25 reps with break between rounds. Vary reps and break time. Or (3) Perform first set of 15 reps, second set of 10 reps, third set of 8 reps, and last set with 5 burpees between each set.

1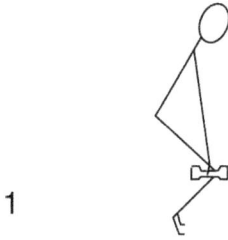

6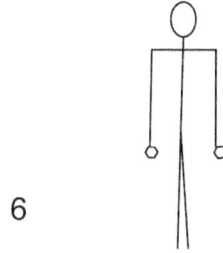

2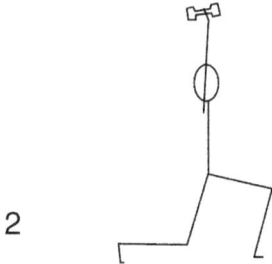

7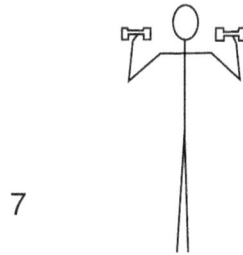

3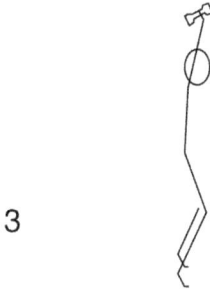

8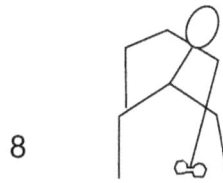

4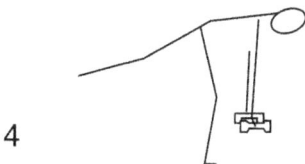

9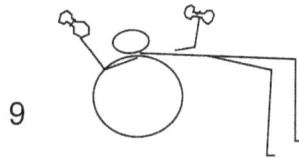

5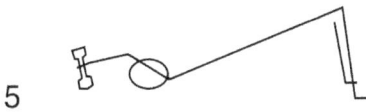

10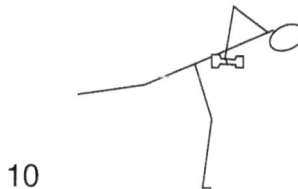

CYBEX® WORKOUT

Leg press machine

Ab crunch machine

Lat pulldown machine

Leg extension machine

Ab twist machine, for obliques

Chest press machine

Leg curl machine

Tricep extension machine

Calf raise machine

Bicep curl machine

Note: Perform (1) first set of 15 reps, (2) second set of 10 reps, (3) third set of 8 reps, and (4) last set with 5 burpees between each set.

DELTOID EXERCISES

Band overhead press

Cable overhead press

Cable raise or fly, including lateral, front and rear

Cable upright row

Dumbbell front raise

Dumbbell overhead press

Dumbbell upright row

Lateral raise machine

Overhead press machine

Stability ball inverted pushup

Note: Perform with fullest range of motion available. Occasionally perform with varying grips and rotations.

EQUALIZER® WORKOUT 1

Wide-grip vertical row on bars

Curl-grip vertical row on bar

Low bridge on flat bar

High bridge on standing bar

180 Wipers up and around bar

Paulinas through and over bar

Wide-grip kneeling tricep extension on bar

Close-grip kneeling tricep extension on bar

Dips on bars

Pushups on bar

Kneeups on bar

Bulgarian lunge, foot on bar to back

Bulgarian lunge, foot on bar to side

Bulgarian lunge, foot on bar to front

Calf raise

FITNESS TIP: Although Calf work is important, it is often overlooked. If adding to your routine, work in slowly as calf muscle will be sore longer and more deeply than most other muscles.

EQUALIZER® WORKOUT 2

Bulgarian squat, one foot on bar

Hip lift, feet on bar, bar may need stabilized by partner
or wall

Hops over low bar

Knee up, hands on bars, dip position

Supine leg circles around bar

Pushup, hands on bar, bar lying on its side

Supine vertical row, hands on bars

Kneeling tricep extension, hands on bar

Supine curl grip vertical row (chin up), hands on bars

Note: Perform (1) first set of 15 reps, (2) second set of 10 reps, (3) third set of 8 reps, and (4) last set with 5 burpees between each set.

FOREARM EXERCISES

Barbell wrist curl

Barbell wrist extension

Cable wrist curl

Cable wrist extension

Dumbbell wrist curl

Dumbbell wrist extension

Grip exercises

Lever exercises

Reverse wrist roller

Wrist roller

Note: Perform with fullest range of motion available.

FREEMOTION® WORKOUT

Squat machine

Ab crunch machine

Lat pulldown machine

Hamstring curl machine

Cobra, back extension cable cross machine

Chest press machine

Hip extension machine

One arm extension machine

Ab twist crunch machine

Bicep curl machine

Note: Perform (1) first set of 15 reps, (2) second set of 10 reps, (3) third set of 8 reps, and (4) last set with 5 burpees between each set.

GLUTE EXERCISES

Birddog kick

Butt blaster

Cable donkey kick

Cable straight leg kick

Deep lunge

Deep squat

Glute machine

Lunge and reach

Squat and reach

Step up

Note: Perform with fullest range of motion available. Avoid hyperextending lumbars.

GWIII'S PRIME-TIME WORKOUT

Bike 5 minutes

Pushups

Situps

Lunges

Seated gray band row

Superman

Squats

Tricep dips on bench

Criss cross

Standing Calf raise with dumbbells

Dumbbell bicep curl

Dumbbell Deadlift

Note: Do 3 sets: First set do 12 reps each exercise, Second set do 20+, Third set do 15 reps. Dedicated to George Whitney III.

HAMSTRING EXERCISES

Deadlift

Forward lunge

Jump lunge

One leg deadlift

Prone dumbbell leg curl

Prone leg curl

Seated leg curl

Standing machine leg curl

Step up

Traveling lunge

Note: Perform with fullest range of motion available. Avoid hyperextending lumbars.

HIP ABDUCTOR EXERCISES

Ankle weight hip abduction

Band hip abduction

Machine hip abduction

Rotary hip machine abduction

Side lying leg raise

Side stepmill with lateral leg extension

Standing cable hip abduction

Step up and lateral kick

Traveling side squat

Versa cuff walking

Note: Perform with fullest range of motion available.

HIP ADDUCTOR EXERCISES

45 degree side lunge

Ankle weight hip adduction

Lateral squat

Machine hip adduction

Rotary Hip machine adduction

Side lying bottom leg lift

Squat and medial cross over kick

Standing cable hip adduction

Step and lateral kick

Wide stance deep squat

Note: Perform with fullest range of motion available. It is not generally recommended to train hip adductors often or heavy.

HIP FLEXOR EXERCISES

Standing bent knee lift

Standing bent knee lift, 45 degree to side

Standing straight leg lift to front

Standing straight leg lift, 45 degrees to side

Supine bent knee lift, alternating legs

Supine bent knee lift, alternating legs

Supine straight leg lift to ceiling

Supine straight leg lift, 45 degrees to side

Supine straight leg lift, alternating legs

Supine straight leg lift, both legs

Note: Perform with fullest range of motion available. The hanging leg raise are great for abs and hip flexors

IRON GYM® WORKOUT 1

Knee in donkey kick, hands on Iron gym on floor

Runners, hands on Iron gym on floor

Half burpees, hands on Iron gym on floor

Straight leg raise, hanging form bar

Back extension, hanging form bar

Bent knee raise, hanging from ab straps

Bicycle, hanging from ab straps

Neutral grip pull up from bar

Pushup, hands on Iron gym on floor

Curl grip chin up from bar, for biceps

Close grip pushup hands on Iron gym on floor

Note: Perform (1) first set of 15 reps, (2) second set of 10 reps, (3) third set of 8 reps, and (4) last set with 5 burpees between each set.

IRON GYM WORKOUT 2

Wide-grip pull up, full body or assisted

Neutral-grip pull up, full body or assisted

Curl-grip chin up, full body or assisted

Pushup, hands on wide-grip

Pushup, hands on neutral-grip

Hanging (strap) straight-leg raise

Hanging (strap) bent-knee raise

Hanging (strap or bar) side swing (obliques)

Running man (strap or bar), stabilize torso and run legs in air

Hanging (strap or bar), back extension (arch) and bent-knee raise

Note: There are numerous exercises that can also be done with iron gym on floor, hooked to bottom of door frame and supine position with bar resting on shin.

MEDICINE BALL WORKOUT

1. Lunge and medicine ball overhead press

2. Squat and medicine ball forward press

3. Standing medicine ball twist

4. Superman with medicine ball in hands

5. Medicine ball mason twist

6. Medicine ball chop

7. Medicine ball situp and throw

8. Pushup with one hand on medicine ball, switch arms

9. Supine medicine ball straight arm pullover

10. Side lunge with medicine ball forward press

11. Jump squat with medicine ball overhead

Note: Perform 2–3 rounds consisting of 30–60 seconds with break between rounds. Vary time and break time.

1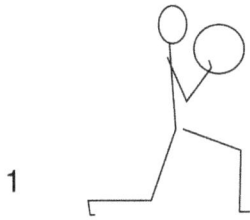

2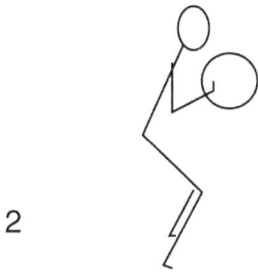

3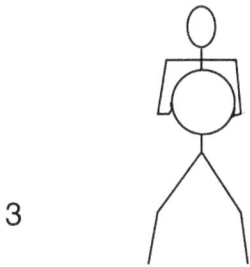

4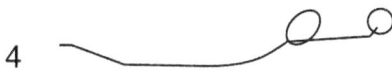

5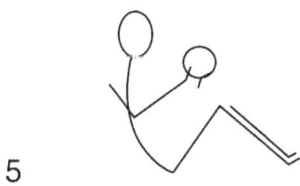

6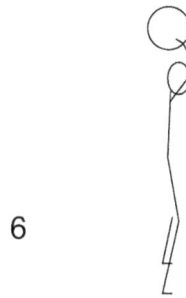

7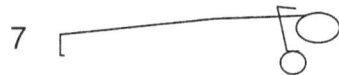

8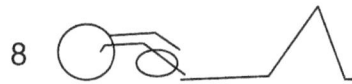

9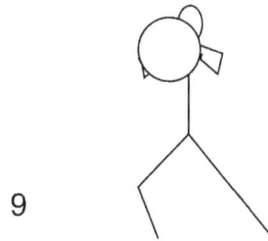

10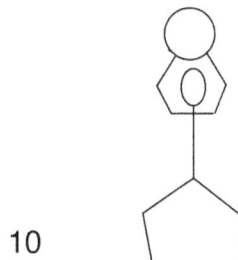

LUMBAR EXERCISES

Birddog

Deadlift

Good morning

Low back machine

Lunge and reach

Roman chair extension

Stability ball prone back extension

Stability ball prone contralateral arm/leg lift

Stability ball prone reverse extension

Superman

Note: Perform with fullest range of motion available.

MAGIC CIRCLE WORKOUT BEGINNER

Squat, circle between knees

Crunch, circle between knees

Hip lift, circle between knees

Situp, circle between hands

Supine inner thigh press, circle between knees

Superman, circle between hands and floor

Standing, circle between hands, press in

Standing, circle behind back between hands

Note: Perform 2 rounds consisting of 10–12 reps with break between rounds. Vary reps and break time.

MAGIC CIRCLE WORKOUT INTERMEDIATE

1. Side lying on forearm, one leg raise, circle between floor and one hand

2. Hip lift circle between knees

3. Squat, circle between knees

4. Supine inner thigh press, circle between knees

5. Crunch, circle between knees

6. Side crunch, circle between ankles

7. Situp, circle between hands

8. Superman, circle between hands and floor

9. Standing, circle behind back between hands

10. Standing overhead press, circle between hands and one hip

Note: Perform 2–3 rounds consisting of 8–16 reps with break between rounds. Vary reps and break time.

1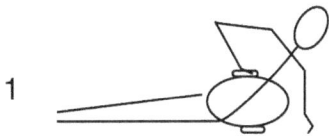

6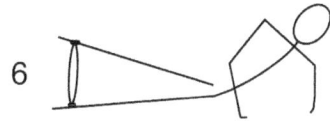

2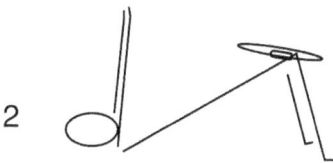

7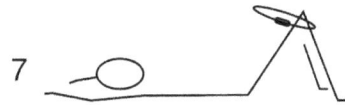

3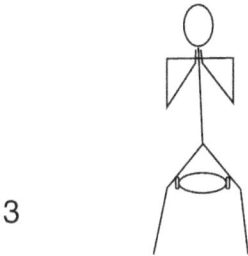

8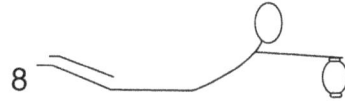

4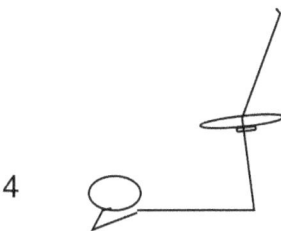

9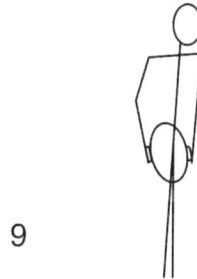

5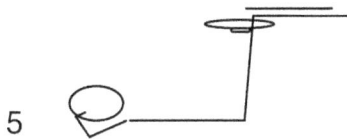

10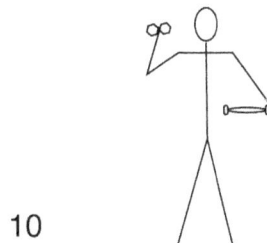

MAGIC CIRCLE WORKOUT ADVANCED

Side leg lift, circle between ankles

Double leg, circle between ankles

Squat, circle between hands

Supine outer thigh press, circle around knees

Roll up, circle between hands

Crisscross with alternating leg in, circle between hands

Teaser, circle between hands

Superman, circle between hands

Hundred, circle between ankles and floor

Saw, circle between hands

Roll over, circle between hands

Paulina, circle between ankles

Floor press, seated, legs wide, circle between hands
and floor

Standing, shoulder abduction, circle around hands,
push out on ring

Overhead press, circle between hands

Chest press, circle between hands

Note: Perform 3–4 rounds consisting of 8–24 reps with break between
rounds. Vary reps and break times.

LYING WORKOUT

Hip lift

One leg bridge

Bicycle

Crunch

Supine spinal twist

Crisscross

Good morning stretch

Superman

Sphinx

Cobra

Up dog

Supine chest fly

Supine tricep extension

Pushup

High plank one arm row

Note: Perform 2–3 rounds consisting of 30–60 seconds with break between rounds. Vary time and break time.

LAT EXERCISES

Assisted pull up machine

Bent over row

Dumbbell pullover

Lat pulldown

Machine pullover

One arm row

Pull up or chin up

Seated low cable row

Seated row machine

Standing straight arm pulldown

Note: Perform with fullest range of motion available. Avoid hyperextending lumbars.

MUSCLE GROUPS TRAINING ORDER BY THOMPSON

Core

Glutes

Lats

Thighs

Chest

Calves

Shoulders

Triceps

Biceps

Forearms

Note: This is a recommended order of priority to train for integrated functionality.

MUSCLE GROUPS TRAINING ORDER BY WEIDER

Legs

Back

Chest

Shoulders

Calves

Upper arms

Forearms

Abdominals

Note: This is a recommended order of priority to train muscle groups for general muscle mass.

Reference: *Ultimate Bodybuilder*, Joe Weider with Bill Reynolds, ©1989, NTC/Contemporary Publishing Group, Inc.

MUSCLES/GROUPS BY SIZE

Gluteals

Quadriceps

Hamstrings

Lats

Pectorals

Abdominals

Erector Spinae

Traps

Calves

FITNESS TIP: Generally it is worthwhile to train muscle groups by size, largest to smallest.

MUSCLES/GROUPS BY STRENGTH

Gluteals

Quadriceps

Hamstrings

Calves

Traps

Lats

Pectorals

Erector Spinae

Triceps

FITNESS TIP: Do daily activities ambidextrously, e.g. brush teeth one day left-handed, one day right.

NECK EXERCISES

Neck extension

Neck flexion

Neck lateral bend

Neck retraction

Neck rotation, full circle

Neck rotation, semi-circle to front

Prone neck extension

Supine neck flexion

Supine neck lateral bend

Supine neck retraction

Note: Perform with proper form and caution.

FITNESS TIP: Understand misuse and overuse to stay safe when training cervicals.

OBLIQUE EXERCISES

Cable side crunch

Dumbbell side bend

High side plank hip lift

Low cable side chop

Machine twist

Prone stability ball twist

Roman chair side lift

Stability ball side crunch

Standing twist

Supine stability ball twist

FITNESS TIP: The core can be thought of as a cube, activating all the muscles in toward the center of the core simultaneously, three-dimensionally.

PILATES WORKOUT

The hundred

The corkscrew

Single leg stretch

Double leg stretch

Single straight leg stretch

Double straight leg stretch

Criss cross

Teaser

The saw

Shoulder bridge

Note: See Chapter 4, Pilates and Yoga Workouts for more details.

POSTERIOR BODYWEIGHT EXERCISES

Bow pose (backbend)

Bridge

Calf raises

Deadlift hands behind head

Lunges for glute

One-leg bridge

One-leg deadlift

Pilates swimmers

Pilates toe squats for hamstring

Prone rear flys

Superdog (quadruped donkey kick) for glute

Superman

Tricep dips

FITNESS TIP: Due to the over-abundance of anterior work, exercise and movement, posterior work is very important for balance, posture and health.

PROPER ROUTINE BUILDING

Be proactive AND reactive

Control powerhouse (core)

Focus on your form and actions (Concentration)

Improve all components (strength, endurance, balance, speed, etc)

Include proper nutrition

Include proper psyche

Include proper recovery periods

Keep routines progressive, functional and integrated

Keep routines varied

Target all muscles

FITNESS TIP: After understanding the fundamentals of fitness, be creative and have fun.

PARTNER ASSISTED TRAINING

Donkey calf raise: partner sitting on top of hips while doing bent-over calf raises

Towel/rope bicep curl

Towel/rope overhead extension

Rope row

Squat with partner on shoulders

Lunge with partner on shoulders

Pushup with partner on back (partner prone)

Supine two-leg ab throw (partner throws legs)

Standing medicine ball twist (partner behind)

Stability ball punches (hold stability ball while partner attempts to punch it out of your grasp

Note: Perform 2–3 rounds consisting of 30–60 seconds with break between rounds. Vary time and break time.

PECTORAL EXERCISES

Barbell bench press

Barbell incline chest press

Cable fly

Chest press machine

Child's pose to Downward dog pose

Dumbbell bench press

Dumbbell incline press

Incline machine chest press

Machine fly

Pec dec

Pushup

Supine pullover

Note: Perform with fullest range of motion available. Avoid hyperextending lumbars.

POWER TRAINING WORKOUT

Power Clean

Clean high pull

Split Jerk

Push jerk

Clean and jerk

Barbell overhead squat

Barbell deadlift

Barbell squat

Barbell chest press

Barbell bent over row

Overhead press

Push press

Barbell snatch

Snatch high pull

Hang clean

FITNESS TIP: For safety and variety, use dumbbells for these movements.

QUADRICEP EXERCISES

Bulgarian lunge

Cable lunge

Cable squat

Forward lunge

Hack squat

Leg extension

Leg press

Squat

Step up

Traveling lunge

Note: Perform with fullest range of motion available. Avoid hyperextending or flexing lumbars.

WORKOUT TRAINING PRINCIPLES BY THOMPSON

Integrated functional training

Isometric training, strength training in which the joint angle and muscle length do not change during contraction

Machine-core supersets, using balance disks in conjunction with machines to engage core muscles

Plyometric training, designed to produce fast, powerful movements, and improve the functions of the nervous system

Posterior training, exercise targeting only the posterior muscles

(continued on next page)

WORKOUT TRAINING PRINCIPLES
BY THOMPSON (Cont.)

Resistance training circuits, high-intensity aerobics using various types of resistance exercises with little or no rest periods

Sequence sets, adding one exercise every circuit without a rest period; up to 10 circuits

Slow-motion training and Speed reps

Total body supersets, a superset consisting of an exercise for each lower body, core, and upper body muscles

Variety training, changing your routine every session

RESISTANCE TRAINING PRINCIPLES BY WEIDER

Compound sets, working opposing muscle groups in back-to-back fashion, taking as little rest as possible in between sets

Continuous Tension, performing each rep of an exercise by never allowing the weight to rest

Muscle priority, training your underdeveloped muscles first

Pre-Exhaust training, pre-fatiguing a larger muscle with a single-joint movement followed by compound movements

Pyramiding, doing first set with less weight for more reps, increasing the weight and finally decreasing the reps again

(continued on next page)

RESISTANCE TRAINING PRINCIPLES BY WEIDER (Cont.)

Set System Training, doing more than one set for each exercise

Split system, split the body parts into two or three sessions and workout two or three times per week

Staggered sets, training smaller body parts like forearms in between all sets for your major body parts

Supersets, alternating two exercises for the same muscle group, taking as little rest as possible between each set

Tri-Sets, doing three sets in a row for the same body part with as little rest as possible in between sets

Reference: *Bodybuilding 101,* ©1995, Robert Wolff, Contemporary Books, Lincolnwood, IL; Wikipedia, Joe Weider, en.wikipediorg/wiki/Joe Weider, November 2009

SEATED WORKOUT

1. Camel pose

2. Boat pose

3. Rabbit pose

4. Hero pose

5. Supine hip lift

6. Mason twist

7. Seated back extension

8. Seated bent over row

9. Seated bent over fly

10. Seated upright row

11. Seated bent over kickback

12. Seated lateral raise

13. Get ups from chair

14. Seated leg extension machine

15. Seated leg curl machine

Note: Perform 2–3 rounds consisting of 30–60 seconds with break between rounds. Vary time and break time.

1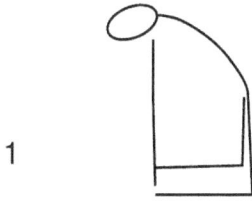

5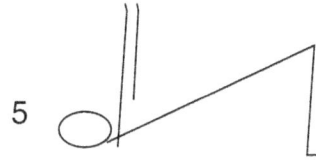

2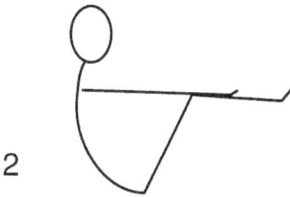

6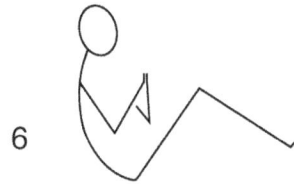

3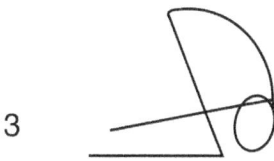

7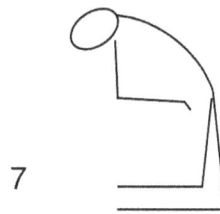

4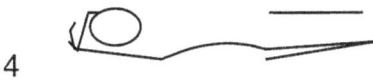

8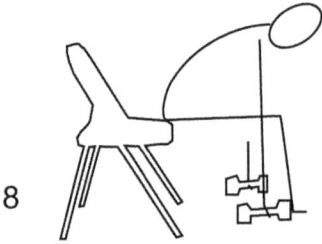

11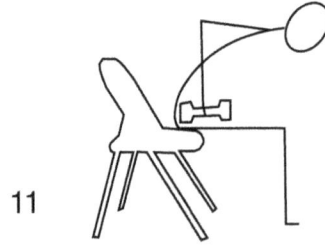

9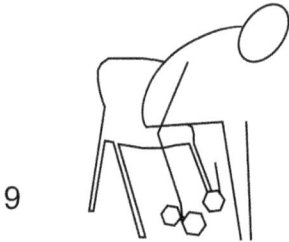

12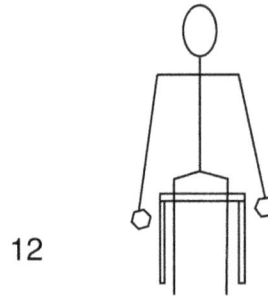

10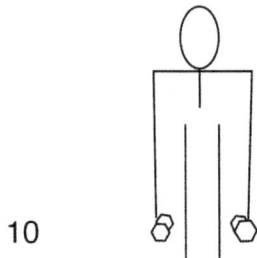

13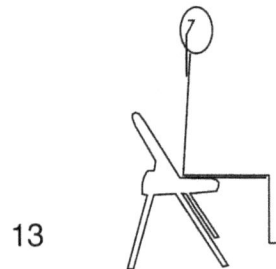

STANDING WORKOUT

Squat

Lunge

Deadlift

Standing calf raise

Twisting side punch

Tae Bo® standing goddess twist

Steam engine, standing alternating knee lift with upper body twist, hands by ears

Standing back extension

Standing arms over twist

Standing side bend

Bent over one arm row

Bent over fly

Upright row, pull elbows up past shoulders

Note: Perform 2–3 rounds consisting of 30–60 seconds with break between rounds. Vary time and break time.

STABILITY BALL WORKOUT BASIC

Wall squat

Wall lunge

Wall calf raise

Crunch

Pushup

Prone back extension/superman

Side crunch

Prone tuck/jackknife

Supine hamstring curl

Rollout with wheel or stability ball

FITNESS TIP: When lunging, assure the knee tracks properly, generally through the second toe line.

STABILITY BALL WORKOUT INTERMEDIATE

Wall squat, stability ball behind low back

Straight leg bridge, stability ball under ankles

One leg wall squat, stability ball behind low back

Supine hip adduction, stability ball between thighs

Supine spinal twist, stability ball under legs

Supine hip abduction, stability ball between thigh and wall

Calf raise, stability ball between abs and wall

Crunch, stability ball under low back

Supine hip lift, stability ball under feet

Birddog, stability ball under torso

Side lying, crunch, stability ball under other side

Back extension, stability ball under torso, hands by ears

(continued on next page)

STABILITY BALL WORKOUT INTERMEDIATE (Cont.)

Skiers, stability ball under knees, shift tuck from side to side

One leg tuck, stability ball under shin

Swimmers, Stability ball under torso, alternating arms

Kneeling butterfly, stability ball under chest

Kneeling row, stability ball under chest

Kneeling, ball side roll, stability ball under hands

Kneeling, alternating arm lift, stability ball under chest

Prone side to side lean, stability ball under hips, legs in air, go from one arm to the other

Pushup, stability ball under shins

Tricep dip, stability ball under hands

Note: Perform 1–3 rounds

STABILITY BALL WORKOUT ADVANCED

Diamond hip lift, feet on stability ball

Supine reverse crunch, hands holding stability ball

Thigh twist, stability ball between ankles, legs in air

Bridge roll, feet on stability ball

Teaser, feet on stability ball

Corkscrew, stability ball between ankles

Side bend, hands by ears, one leg straight, stability ball under hips

Pike stand or swimmers

Pushup, alternating leg lift, stability ball under feet

Twist, stability ball under waist, arms out stretched

Alternating leg raise, stability ball under shins

Leg extension, stability ball under hips

(continued on next page)

STABILITY BALL WORKOUT ADVANCED (Cont.)

Pushup, stability ball under feet

Prone scissors, on forearms, stability ball under hips

Tricep dip, feet on stability ball

Twist in bridge, stability ball under shoulders

Boat on stability ball

Backstroke, stability ball under rib cage

V sit on stability ball

Twist crunch, stability ball under mid back, alternate knee lift

Standing split, stability ball under hands

Bulgarian lunge, stability ball under one foot

Side squat, stability ball under one foot

Note: Perform 2–4 rounds.

SWIM STROKES

Backstroke

Breast stroke

Butterfly

Crawl

Elementary backstroke

Inverted breast stroke

Overarm side stroke

Sidestroke

Trudgen crawl

Note: As with all fitness, proper posture and form is key. Consult Alexander Technique for details on proper functional posturing.

TAI CHI/QIGONG MOVEMENTS

Chinese drum (torso twist)

Toe touch arm lift (arm raise)

Opening the chest (chest expansion)

Painting a rainbow

Separating the clouds

Rotating the arms in a horse-riding stance (shoulder rotation)

Rowing a boat in the middle of a lake (upward rowing)

Carry Ball in front of the shoulders

Gazing at the moon

Turning the waist and pushing with the palm

FITNESS TIP: Qigong has many benefits, two of which are physical and mental recovery.

TIBIALIS ANTERIOR (SHIN) EXERCISES

Any above exercises with one-leg only

Standing on step toe lift, two leg

Standing on step toe lift, single leg

Seated toe lift

Seated, legs straight, band around toes, toe lift (dorsiflexion)

Seated, legs straight, toe lift (dorsiflexion)

Standing toe lift

FITNESS TIP: The shin muscle are important to foot and leg health and should not be neglected in training.

TRAPEZIUS EXERCISES

Barbell bent over row

Barbell front raise

Barbell shrug

Barbell upright row

Cable shrug

Deadlift

Dumbbell shrug

Dumbbell upright row

One arm cable shrug

Shrug machine

Note: Perform with fullest range of motion available. Heavy deadlift must only be performed by experienced lifters.

TRICEP EXERCISES

Assisted tricep dip machine

Bench tricep dip

Cable overhead tricep extension

Cable press down

Close grip chest press

Close grip pushup

Overhead dumbbell extension

Roman chair tricep dip

Supine overhead tricep extension

Tricep extension machine

Note: Perform with fullest range of motion available.

TWENTY'S WORKOUT

20 pullups

20 weighted squats

20 teasers

20 chinups

20 weighted lunges

20 wheel rollouts

20 pushups with light-weight person on back

20 weighted calf raises

20 weighted supermen

20 weighted tri dips

20 deadlifts

20 side crunches

Note: Repeat 3 times. Only perform pushups if correct form can be kept.

WORKOUT BASICS

Continuous breathing, exhale on exertion

Do slow controlled reps, usually between

Exercise all muscle groups unless contraindicated

Focus on exercise

Maintain neutral spine/pelvis as appropriate

Perform 8 and 20 per set

Stretch between sets

Take one-to-two recovery days per week

Train unilaterally and asymmetrically (train more on the side of your body that is weaker either in strength or in balance)

Use multiple and single joint movements (multiple joint movements use more than one joint such as pushups; single joint movements use one joint such as chest flys)

Use variety and train core

FITNESS TIP: One of the keys to breath, is to always keep breath moving, not holding.

WORKOUT SEQUENCE

Warm-up

Traditional stretching

Resistance training for the major muscles

Training for minor muscles

Balance training

Functionally integrated training

Core training

Power and speed-agility-quickness training

Cool down

Self-myofascial release

FITNESS TIP: Think outside the box to find the exercises that work best for you.

WORKOUT TRAINING HAZARDS

Barbell behind neck press

Bench press without spotter

Deep knee flexion

Heavy back squat/Heavy squat without spotters

Heavy behind neck pulldown

Heavy standing bent arm rotation

Losing focus

Overhead press without spotter

Plyometric Smith machine bench press

Standing stability ball overhead press

FITNESS TIP: Use gloves or talc when needed.

"YOGA" WORKOUT BASIC

Chair

Downward facing dog

Extended side angle

Humble warrior

Intense side stretch

Lizard

Mountain

Revolved triangle

Warrior I

Wide stance forward fold

Note: Perform with fullest range of motion available, let breath increase muscle and energy length.

"YOGA" WORKOUT INTERMEDIATE

Chair with overhead dumbbell tricep extension

Downdog with alternating leg raise

Downdog with alternating dumbbell lat row

Forward fold with alternating leg raise

Half forward fold with dumbbell rear deltoid fly

Hi lunge or warrior stance with dumbbell shoulder side raise

High lunge or warrior stance with dumbbell bicep curl

Mountain with dumbbell overhead shoulder press

Plank with alternating dumbbell lat row

Scorpion

Note: Add burpees, half burpees, runners, mountain climbers to plank pose for add difficulty or cardio.

"YOGA" WORKOUT ADVANCED

surya namaskara A, holding dumbbell

Dumbbell bent over fly

Dumbbell front raise

Dumbbell bent over kickback

Dumbbell hammer curl

Dumbbell bent over row, neutral grip

Dumbbell overhead press

Dumbbell bent over row, pronated grip

High plank leg raise

Superman dumbbell arm raise

Superman with leg laterals

Superman with dumbbell arm laterals

Scorpion

Pushups

chaturanga

Up dog

Down dog

Revolved down dog

surya namaskara B, holding dumbbell throughout class.

Note: May be performed without weights

"YOGA" WORKOUT EXTENDED

surya namaskara A, holding dumbbell

Dumbbell bent over fly

Dumbbell front raise

Dumbbell bent over kickback

Dumbbell hammer curl

Dumbbell bent over row, neutral grip

Dumbbell overhead press

Dumbbell bent over row, pronated grip

Dumbbell upright row

Dumbbell bent over row, supinated grip

Dumbbell overhead press, pronated grip

Dumbbell bent over kickback, supinated grip

High plank leg raise

(continued on next page)

"YOGA" WORKOUT EXTENDED (Cont.)

Superman dumbbell arm raise

Superman with leg laterals

Superman with dumbbell arm laterals

Scorpion

Leg curl

Superman contralateral lifts

Runners and Half burpees

Pushups

chaturanga

Up dog and Down dog

Revolved down dog

High lunge dumbbell bicep curl

High lunge dumbbell lateral raise

High lunge dumbbell overhead press

High lunge dumbbell outstretched

surya (no 3) namaskara B, holding dumbbell

FITNESS TIP: See Chapter 4, Pilates and Yoga Workouts for more details.

CHAPTER 3

Rehabilitation & Recovery Workouts

PHYSICAL REHABILITATION is a system of exercises, manipulations, and other methods designed to restore or improve motor skills to a functional level.

ACTIVE RECOVERY or "active rest" is a hybrid between resting and exercising. It involves purposely exercising in a specialized fashion or a low-intensity as a means of helping your body recover from competition, high-intensity exercise, or muscle soreness. And a growing body of research shows that active recovery is more beneficial than passive recovery, completely resting from exercise. www.sparkpeople.com/blog/blog.asp?post=fitness_defined_active_and_passive_recovery)

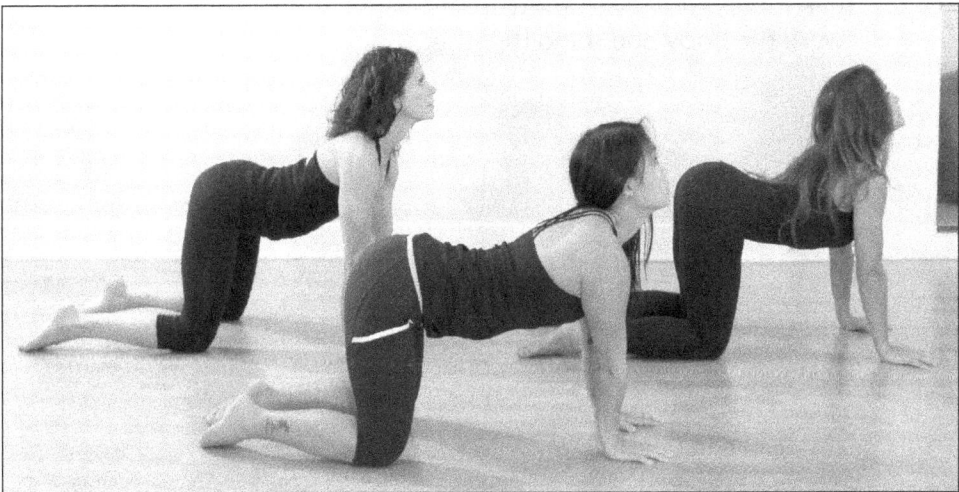

Cow pose

AGILITY TRAINING

Agility ring drills

Change direction and speed drills

Cone drills

Hurdle drills

Ladder drills

Proprioceptive drills (spatial awareness)

Simultaneous speed and balance drills

Shuttle drills

Tire drills

Any combination of the above

FITNESS TIP: Coordination and spatial awareness are important aspects of training that when done properly work the body and mind together.

AQUATIC TRAINING

Aquatic cross training, land and water exercise intervals

Butterfly laps

Deep water lunging

Laps without using arms

Laps without using legs

Speed strokes

Surface diving drills

Water Pilates

Water Tai Chi

Water yoga

FITNESS TIP: Aquatic training has many therapy and recovery effects.

BAND TRAINING

Squat, band under feet

Lunge, band under foot

Calf raise, band under toes

Crunch, band anchored behind and over shoulders

Pushup, band in one hand, twist and lift one arm after each pushup

Bicep curl, band under feet

Bent-over row/anchored low row

Overhead tricep extension, band under feet

Standing straight-arm swing, band anchored in front, high

Standing rear fly, band anchored in front, chest level

FITNESS TIP: Check bands regularly for cracks and loss of integrity and immediate dispose and replace those needed.

BALANCE TRAINING

Bosu® ball training

Cable exercises

Drills on disks, boards and foam

Line walking and variations

Lunge and variations

Medicine ball drills

One-leg training

Plyometric training

Stability ball training

Any combination of the above

FITNESS TIP: Bosu ball are an integral part of fitness, with many uses including balance, stability, strength, coordination and agility.

COORDINATION TRAINING

Agility training exercises

Contra-lateral movements

Double Bosu® jumps

Exercises with one or both eyes closed

Juggling

Ladder drills

Lower Body plyometric exercises

Medicine ball throws on Bosu® ball

Plyometric medicine ball exercises, throwing off wall

Plyometric medicine ball exercises, throwing to partner

FITNESS TIP: Coordination is a great way to train mind and body together.

CALISTHENIC TRAINING

Back Lunge

Handstand

Jump squat

Lunge

Lying leg raise

Pullup/Chinup

Pushup

Situp

Squat

Squat and thrust

FITNESS TIP: Calisthenics are a valuable yet underutilized part of fitness.

COOLING DOWN BASICS

Align your energy with Tai chi or Qigong movements such as the wheel

Check in, mentally think what a good workout you had and how now you will cool down and recover

Keep moving lightly, stopping right after exercise is not recommended

Mild Sun salutations work great for cool downs

Perform stretches, particularly for the muscles groups exercised

Refuel, drink water or a shake as required

Stay warm, do not cool the muscles too soon

Take full continual breaths

Walk on treadmill or other cardio machine at very low level

FITNESS TIP: Lying in savasana is a wonderful method of recovery.

ESSENTIALS FOR OPTIMUM SLEEPING

A regular waking and sleeping schedule

Clean Bedding

Comfortable mattress and pillow

Daily exercise but not just before bedtime

Dark, cool, quiet room

Little or no heavy or spicy foods before bedtime

Reasonably early dinner

Relaxed state of mind

Stimulant free body

Reference: *The Only 127 Things You Need: A Guide to Life's Essentials,* Donna Wilkinson, Penguin Group, New York, ©2008

FASTING BENEFITS

Fasting Promotes Detoxification

Fasting Improves Insulin Sensitivity

Fasting Rests Digestive System

Fasting Boosts Immunity

Fasting Corrects High Blood Pressure

Fasting May Help to Overcome Addictions

Fasting Promotes Weight Loss

Fasting Resolves Inflammatory Response

Fasting Promotes Healthy Diet

Fasting Clears the Skin and Whitens the Eyes

Source: www.wonderslist.com/10-health-benefits-of-fasting/

Note: Fasting is a good practice, if properly implemented. It promotes elimination of toxins from the body, reduces blood sugar and fat stores. It promote healthy eating habits and boost immunity. Research suggests there are major health benefits of fasting to caloric restriction.

HIP REHAB WORKOUT BASIC

Supine bridge

Supine hip adduction, ball or pillow between thighs, push in and hold

Supine pelvic tilt

Supine hip abduction, move legs out and in

Supine hip flexion, lift leg up and down

Side lying hip abduction, lift top leg up and down

Side lying hip adduction, lift bottom leg up and down

Seated leg extension, lift one leg and hold

Seated two leg extension isometric

Note: Perform more work on hip that is weaker, less flexible, etc.

HIP REHAB WORKOUT INTERMEDIATE

Supine heel slides

Supine bridge

Supine snow angel

Ankle pumps

Ankle circles

Ankle extension/flexion

Ankle alphabet

Seated marching, regular

Seated marching, high knees

Seated arm circles

Seated reverse arm circles

Seated side bend

Seated upper cut punching

Note: Perform more work on hip that is weaker, less flexible, etc.

HIP REHAB WORKOUT ADVANCED

Supine double heel slides

Supine one leg hip lift

Supine snow angel

Ankle pumps

Standing ankle circles

Standing ankle extension/flexion

Standing ankle alphabet

Standing marching, regular

Standing marching, high knees

Standing arm circles

Standing reverse arm circles

Standing side bend

Standing upper cut punching

Standing non-ballistic butt kickers, marching
and kick foot toward glute

Note: Perform more work on hip that is weaker, less flexible, etc.

HIP WORKOUT STATIC

Standing cross ankle side bend

Standing quad stretch, pull foot to glute

Wide leg runner's stretch (similar to lizard pose)

Standing hip stretch, ankle on opposite thigh, lean forward, may hold chair or table for support

Standing hamstring stretch, heel on step, lean forward

Toe touch

Note: For traditional static stretches to be effective, determine the correct muscle angle (function) and vary the stretch duration from 2–60 seconds

LUMBAR SCOLIOSIS WORKOUT

Prone pose

Sphinx pose

Up dog pose

Standing back extension

Supine knee in

Seated back flexion

Standing back flexion

Note: Use the convex side for strengthening or lean toward the convex area for flexibility as directed. Based on the McKenzie Method.

LUMBAR FLEX

Single knee to chest

Knees to chest

Supine straight leg to chest

Supine single knee spinal twist, arms out

Supine spinal twist, arms out

Supine single knee spinal twist, arm assisted

Note: Do 2–6 rounds of 20–120 seconds

RANGE OF MOTION UPPER BODY

Head tilts, forward and back

Head tilts, side to side

Head turns

Shoulder movement, up and down

Shoulder movement, side to side

Shoulder rotation

Elbow bends

Wrist bends

Wrist rotation

Palm up, palm down

Finger bends

Finger spreads

Finger-to-thumb touches

Thumb-to-palm stretches

Source: www.drugs.com/cg/active-range-of-motion-exercises.html

RANGE OF MOTION LOWER BODY

Hip and knee bends

Leg lifts

Leg movement, side to side.

Leg rotation, in and out

Knee rotation, in and out

Ankle bends.

Ankle rotation

Toe bends

Toe spreads

Source: www.drugs.com/cg/active-range-of-motion-exercises.html

Note: Active range of motion exercises help improve joint function. Range of motion is how far you can move your joints in different directions. These exercises help you move each joint through its full range of motion. Movement can help keep your joints flexible, reduce pain, and improve balance and strength.

RECOVERY BASICS

At least 30 minutes per day downtime, self-time, no worries

Consultation with health practitioner for injuries lasting over 14 days

Deep sleep of proper duration

Elimination or moderation of alcohol, caffeine, and other diuretics

One day off per week and one week off per quarter

Proper nutrition including breakfast and easily assimilated multi-vitamin/mineral source

Reduction of medication as per practitioner

Regular flexibility including Pilates/Yoga

Regular massage

Sufficient hydration

FITNESS TIP: Massage therapy can not only treat issues it is great as a diagnostic tool as well.

RECOVERY DRINKS

Almond milk

Ayurvedic electrolyte drink

Coconut milk

Coconut water

Combo shake (proteins, carbs and fats)

Fruit shake

Protein shake

Veggie shake

Water

Fitness Note: All ingredients should be whole and organic.

RECOVERY FOODS

Avocado

Bananas

Berries

Broccoli

Coconut Oil

Garlic

Ginger

Green Tea

Pineapple

Salmon

Note: When you do strenuous exercise your body starts to produce inflammation to help protect your muscle and joints. While this level of inflammation is healthy and normal it is important to ensure you allow your body to recover correctly after workouts.

Source: http://truegymfitness.com/top-10-recovery-foods/

RECOVERY WORKOUTS

Cycling

Hiking

Lighter Weight Lifting

Self-myofascial release (SMR)

Swimming

Walking

Yoga

Source: www.builtlean.com/2013/01/21/active-recovery-workout-ideas/

FITNESS TIP: Often low back pain originates from the shoulders or hips.

S-I JOINT STRETCHES

Camel

Childs

Cowface

Extended side angle

Lizard

Low lunge

Pigeon

Seated forward fold

Supine eagle legs

Triangle

FITNESS TIP: When treating tight S-I joints, also look at tightness in the opposite hip flexor area.

S-I JOINT WORKOUT BASIC

Lying eagle legs

Seated forward fold pose

Camel pose

Childs pose

Triangle pose

Extended side angle pose

Low lunge pose

Lizard pose

Note: Lumbar caution with too wide or too close stances; Knee caution with pigeon, king pigeon, double pigeon; cowface poses. Strengthen area with cobra, locust, airplane, bow poses.

S-I JOINT WORKOUT INTERMEDIATE

Reclined angle pose (lying butterfly)

Sphinx pose

Childs pose

Lying eagle legs

Childs pose

Pigeon pose

Childs pose

Lizard pose

Childs pose

Cowface pose

Childs pose

Hero pose

Childs pose

Note: Lumbar caution with too wide or too close stances; Knee caution with pigeon, king pigeon, double pigeon; cowface poses. Strengthen area with cobra, locust, airplane, bow poses.

S-I JOINT WORKOUT ADVANCED

Reclined angle pose (lying butterfly)

Sphinx pose

Lying eagle legs

Childs pose

Lying spinal twist

Seated spinal twist

Childs pose

Pigeon pose

Lizard pose

Childs pose

Kneeling split

Threaded plank, straight-leg pigeon

Childs pose

Cowface pose

Hero pose

Childs pose

Note: Lumbar caution with too wide or too close stances; Knee caution with pigeon, king pigeon, double pigeon; cowface poses. Strengthen area with cobra, locust, airplane, bow poses.

S-I JOINT WORKOUT PROGRESSION

Childs pose

Sphinx pose

Childs pose

Lying eagle legs

Seated forward fold pose

Reclined angle pose (lying butterfly)

Camel pose

Cowface pose

Hero pose

Pigeon pose

Low lunge pose

Lizard pose

Triangle pose

Extended side angle pose

Childs pose

Note: Lumbar caution with too wide or too close stances; Knee caution with pigeon, king pigeon, double pigeon; cowface poses. Strengthen area with cobra, locust, airplane, bow poses.

SCOLIOSIS YOGA WORKOUT

1. Mountain pose

2. Tree Pose

3. Triangle Pose

4. Boat Pose

5. Child Pose

6. Cat/Cow

7. Side lying crunch on left side, bottom arm on floor

8. Superman, lift right arm and left leg

9. Side lying crunch on left side, bottom arm across chest

10. Cobra Pose, lift right shoulder

Note: For C-curve, thoracic convex on right side work that side more and stretch left side more.

1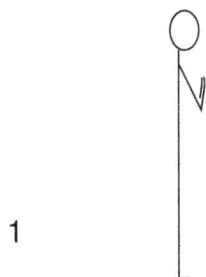

2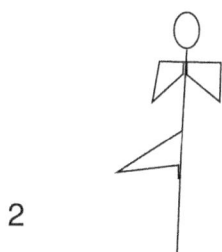

3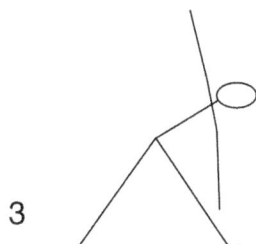

4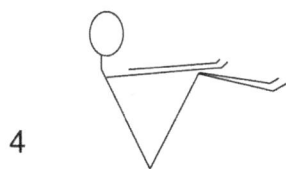

5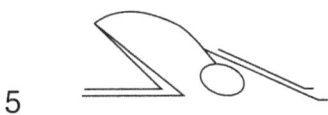

6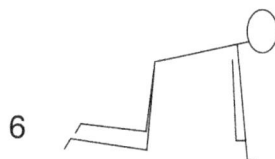

7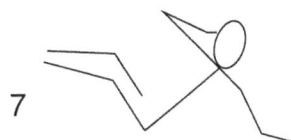

8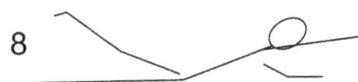

9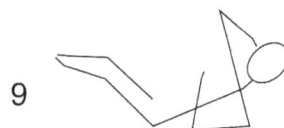

10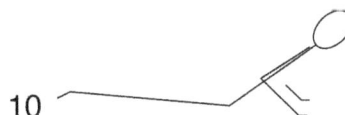

SCOLIOSIS MYOROLLER WORKOUT

Scorpions

Seated side bend to right over myoroller

Standing side bend to left

Supine myoroller bicycle

Supine myoroller crunch

Supine myoroller march

Supine spinal twist, both knees to right

Supine spinal twist, right knee to left

Supine straight leg twist, right leg to left

Supine upper body twist to right

Note: Exercises are designed for S-curve: cervical convex left, thoracic convex right, lumbar convex left. Qigong and Myofascial release are also very beneficial.

CHAPTER 4

Pilates & Yoga Workouts

PILATES is a physical fitness system that focuses on the core postural muscles with help keep the body balanced and which are essential to providing support to the spine. Pilates exercises teach the awareness of breath, alignment of the spine and aim to strengthen the deep torso muscles. (synergywellness4u .com/resources)

YOGA is a healing system of theory and practice. It is a combination of breathing exercises, physical postures, and meditation that has been practiced for more than 5,000 years. (en.wikipedia.org)

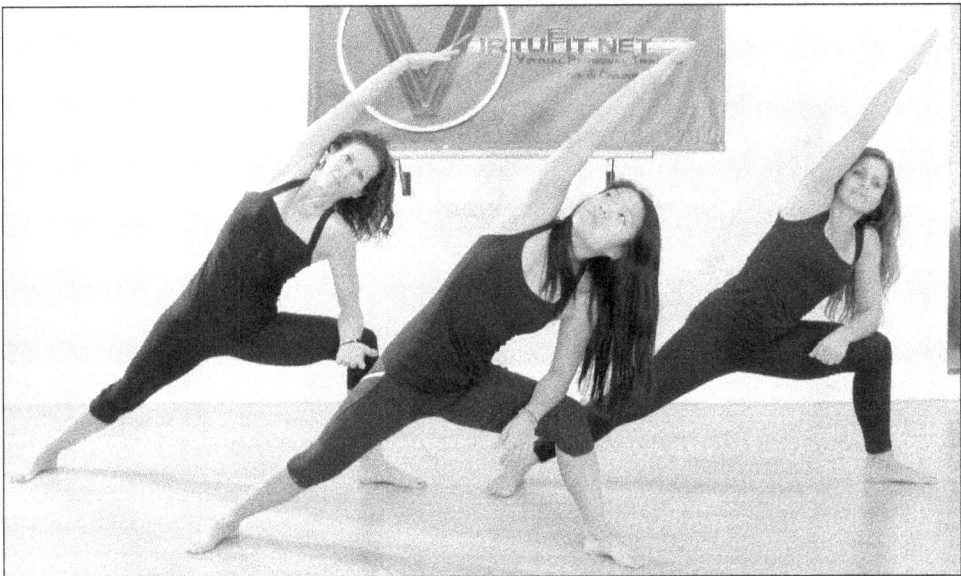

Modified triangle pose

ASHTANGA YOGA

Sun Salutation A/B

Mountain pose

Forward fold pose (2 poses)

Triangle pose

Revolved triangle pose

Extended side angle pose

Revolved side angle pose

Wide leg forward fold (4 poses)

Side intense stretch pose

Extended hand to big toe

Half lotus intense stretch pose

Chair pose

Warrior I/II

Seated staff pose

Seated forward fold (2 poses)

Incline plane pose

One leg forward fold pose (3 poses)

(continued on next page)

ASHTANGA YOGA (Cont.)

One knee up forward fold pose

Seated spinal twist pose

Boat pose/Boat handstand pose

Crow pose

Tortoise pose

Bound angle pose

Wide angle forward fold (3 poses)

Reclining big toe pose (2 poses)

Plow, both big toes pose

Upward facing pose

Plow, both big toes pose

Wheel pose

Shoulder stand pose

3Plow pose

Ear pressure pose

Fish pose

Tripod headstand pose

savasana

GLOBAL YOGA RETREATS

Bahia, Brasil – Butterfly House Bahia

Boracay Island, Philippines – Mandala Spa and Villas

Gstaad, Switzerland – Formentera Yoga

Kerala, India – The Leela

Koh Samui, Thailand – Absolute Sanctuary

Lombardy, Italy – L'Albereta

Marrakech, Morocco – Dar Justo

Sussex, UK – Ockenden Manor Hotel & Spa

Turks & Caicos, Caribbean – Parrot Cay by COMO

Utah, USA – Amangiri

Note: If you fancy unrolling your yoga mat somewhere a little more exciting than your local studio, check out our selection of yoga retreats taking place around the world over the coming months. From Brazil to Boracay and beyond, there's plenty on offer to suit everybody—from less-bendy beginners, through to asana experts.

Source: www.insignia-lb.com/2014/02/03/top-10-yoga-retreats/

HIP SEATED YOGA

Seated forward fold pose

Wide leg forward fold pose

Half lotus pose

Pigeon pose

King pigeon pose

Double pigeon pose

Cow face pose

Note: Perform 2–3 rounds holding for 20–60 seconds. Perform more on side needed. Vary time and sequence.

HIP STANDING YOGA

Standing forward fold pose

Wide leg forward fold pose

Triangle pose

Side angle pose

Low lunge pose

Lizard pose

King pigeon pose

Note: Perform 2–3 rounds holding for 20–60 seconds. Perform more on side needed. Vary time and sequence.

HIP YOGA PROGRESSION

Seated forward fold pose

Wide leg forward fold pose

Half lotus pose

Pigeon pose

King pigeon pose

Double pigeon pose

Cow face pose

Standing forward fold pose

Wide leg forward fold pose

Triangle pose

Side angle pose

Low lunge pose

Lizard pose

Standing ankle on thigh, hold onto bar and lower hips

Note: Perform 2–3 rounds holding for 20–60 seconds. Perform more on side needed. Vary time and sequence.

HOT YOGA

Standing deep breathing

Half moon pose

Awkward pose

Eagle pose

Standing head to knee pose

Dancer pose

Warrior III

Standing separate leg stretching pose

Triangle pose

Standing separate leg, head to knee pose

Tree pose

Toe stand pose

savasana

Wind removing pose

Situp with double exhale

(continued on next page)

HOT YOGA (Cont.)

Cobra pose

Locust pose

Full locust pose

Bow pose

Fixed firm pose (hero)

Half tortoise pose

Camel pose

Rabbit pose

Separate leg stretching head to knee pose

Spine twisting pose

Blowing in firm pose

Note: Temperature is generally about 100 degrees Fahrenheit (38 Celsius).

INTRO YOGA 1

Accomplished pose

Balanced table pose

Balanced bound angle pose

Belly twist A pose

Belly twist B pose

Boat pose

Bound angle pose

Bow pose

Bridge pose

Camel pose

Cat tilt pose

Chair pose

Chair twist pose

Child pose

Cobra pose

Corpse pose

Cow face pose

Crab pose (reverse table pose)

Crane pose

Crescent pose

INTRO YOGA 2

Crocodile pose

Dancer pose

Dog tilt pose

Dolphin pose

Down dog pose

Head to toe pose

Down frog pose

Eagle pose

Easy pose

Eight limb pose

Extended dog pose

Extended hand to toe pose

Extended leg squat pose

Extended side angle pose

Supine extended hand to toe pose

Firelog pose

Fish pose

Flowering lotus pose

Full lotus pose

Garland pose

INTRO YOGA 3

Gate pose

Goddess pose

Gracious pose

Half bound lotus forward fold pose

Half bound lotus pose

Half bow pose

Half camel pose

Half circle pose

Half forward fold pose

Half locust pose

Half lord of fish A pose

Half lord of fish B pose

Half lotus pose

Half moon pose

Half prayer twist pose

Half pyramid pose

Half shoulder stand pose

Half hero pose

Half up seated pose

Half wind relieving pose

INTRO YOGA 4

Head to toe pose

Hero pose

High lunge pose

High plank pose

Inclined plane pose

Joyful baby pose

Lion pose

Locust pose

Low plank pose

Low warrior I

One handed tiger pose

One leg boat pose

One leg bridge pose

One leg down dog pose

One leg king pigeon pose

Plow pose

Prayer squat pose

Praycr twist pose

Pyramid pose

Rabbit pose

INTRO YOGA 5

Revolved down dog pose

Revolved half moon pose

Revolved head to knee pose

Revolved side angle pose

Revolved triangle pose

Seated angle pose

Seated forward fold pose

Seated head to knee pose

Seated head to toe pose

Seated split pose

Seated yoga seal pose

Side seated angle pose

Snake pose

Sphinx pose

Staff pose

Standing backbend pose

Standing forward fold pose

Standing head to knee pose

Standing split pose

Standing yoga seal pose

INTRO YOGA 6

Star pose

Table pose

Threading the needle pose

Tiger pose

Tiptoe pose

Tortoise pose

Tree pose

Triangle pose

Up dog pose

Upright seated angle pose

Upward forward fold pose

Warrior I

Warrior II

Warrior III

Warrior seal

Wide leg forward bend pose

Note: Intro classes of this nature are intended merely to introduce a student to asana, not the entire yoga flow.

MOON SALUTATION 1

Mountain pose, raised arms

Crescent moon pose

Goddess pose

Star pose

Triangle pose

Pyramid pose

High lunge pose

Forward facing lunge pose

Yoga squat pose

Forward facing lunge pose

High lunge pose

Pyramid pose

Triangle pose

Star pose

Goddess pose

Standing side bend pose

Crescent moon pose

Mountain pose, raised arms

MOON SALUTATION 2

Mountain pose, prayer

Mountain pose, raised arms

Standing forward fold pose

Prayer squat pose

Crescent lunge pose

High lunge pose

Half moon pose

Extended child pose

Cobra pose

Extended child pose

Half moon pose

High lunge pose

Crescent lunge pose

Prayer squat pose

Standing forward fold pose

Mountain pose, raised arms

Mountain pose, prayer

MOON SALUTATION 3

Mountain pose, raised arms

Standing forward fold, hand to foot

High lunge pose, Equestrian

Crescent Lunge pose, Lord Hanuman

Extended child pose, pose of the moon

High lunge pose, Equestrian

Crescent Lunge pose, Lord Hanuman

Cobra pose

Extended child pose, Pose of the moon

Half moon pose, Pose of the moon

Prayer squat pose

Mountain pose, prayer

Note: Moon Salutations, also known as chandra namaskar, are a soothing yet empowering variation and counterbalance to classical Sun Salutations (surya namaskar). They allow us to honor the yin or feminine side of our energy, in contrast to the Sun Salutations, which are more yang, or masculine, in nature.

Source: www.eternity-yoga.com and www.proliberty.com/pranayoga/ChandraNamaskar.html

MEGA YOGA FLOW PART 1

Mountain

Standing backbend

Crescent

Star

Chair

Chair twist

Goddess

Prayer squat

Garland

Tiptoe

Extended leg squat

Half forward fold

Forward fold

Standing yoga seal

Up forward fold

Wide leg for bend

Headstand prep

Crane

Mountain

Tree

(continued on next page)

MEGA YOGA FLOW PART 1 (Cont.)

Shiva

Ext. hand to toe

Eagle

Dancer

Standing head to knee

Half bound lotus

Forward fold

Standing splits

Half moon

Revolved half moon

Warrior III

Pyramid

Revolved triangle

Triangle

Low warrior I

Half prayer twist

Half pyramid

High lunge

Warrior I

(continued on next page)

MEGA YOGA FLOW PART 1 (Cont.)

Warrior II

Warrior seal

Revolved side angle

Extended side angle A

Prayer twist

Revolved warrior

Mountain

Down dog

One leg down dog

Revolved Down

Dog

Eight limb

High plank

Staff

Down frog

Low plank

Dolphin

Hero

Half circle

Gate & Camel

MEGA YOGA FLOW PART 2

Lion

Cat tilt

Dog Tilt

Table

Tiger

Balance table

One handed tiger

Extended dog

Rabbit

Thread the needle

Seated yoga seal

Crocodile

Sphinx

Cobra

Up dog

Half locust

Locust

Snake

Half bow

Bow

(continued on next page)

MEGA FLOW YOGA PART 2 (Cont.)

Staff posture

Easy

Bound angle

Accomplished

Gracious

Half lotus

Full lotus

Half lord of fish A

Half lord of fish B

One leg boat

Half up seated angle

Boat

Bal. bound angle

Flowering lotus

Up seated angle

Seated forward bend

Seated head to knee

One leg king pig

Cow face

(continued on next page)

MEGA FLOW YOGA PART 2 (Cont.)

Rev. head to knee

Side seated angle

Tortoise

Seated angle

Seated splits

Bridge

One leg bridge

Incline plane

Crab

Wheel

Half shoulder stand

Plow

Supine bound angle

Half hero

Hero

Fish

Wind

Half wind

Supine pigeon

Joyful baby & Corpse

NOTABLE YOGA TEACHERS

A.G. Mohan and Indra, Svastha Yoga

Ana Forrest, Forrest yoga

B.K.S. Iyengar, Iyengar Yoga

Baron Baptiste, Power Yoga

Beth Shaw, YogaFit

Bikram Choudhury, Bikram Yoga

David Life and Sharon Gannon, Jivamukti Yoga

John Friend, Anusara Yoga

Lakshmi Voelker, Chair Yoga

Lilias Folan, "First Lady" of Western Yoga

Rodney Yee

Shiva Rea, yoga chant and dance

Sri K. Pattabhi Jois, Ashtanga Yoga

Sri T. Krishnamacharya

T.K.V. Desikachar Krishnamacharya, Yoga Mandiram

Wai Lana

PILATES BASIC

1. Hundred

2. Roll up

3. Leg circles

4. Rolling like a ball

5. Single leg stretch

6. Straight leg stretch

7. Spine stretch

8. Saw

9. Single leg kick

10. Modified bridge

11. Modified swimmers

12. Seal

Note: Pilates is designed with generally low rep schemes.

1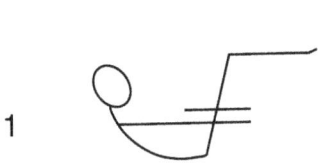

7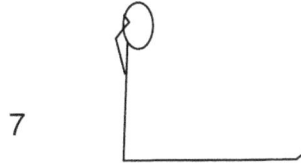

8

2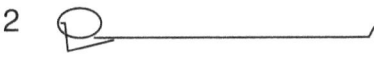

3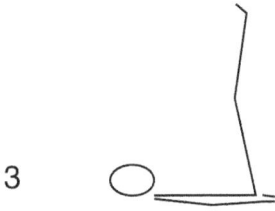

9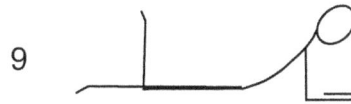

4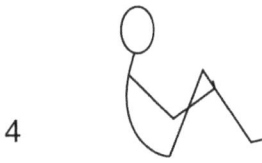

10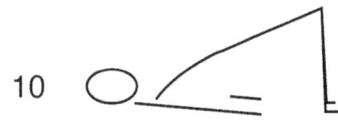

5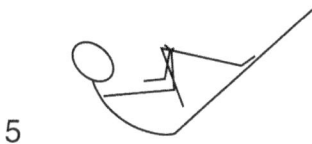

11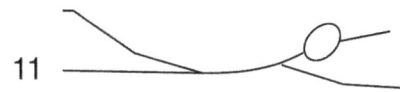

6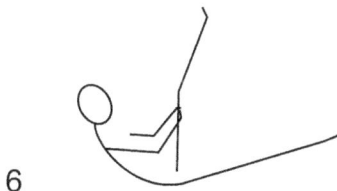

12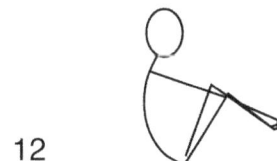

PILATES INTERMEDIATE

Hundred

Roll up

Roll over

Single leg circle

Rolling like a ball

Single leg stretch

Double leg stretch

Straight leg stretch

Double straight leg stretch

Crisscross

Spine stretch

Open leg balance and rocker

Corkscrew

Saw

Single leg kick

Double leg kick

Neck pull

Modified bridge

Teasers

Swimmers

Seal

Modified pushups

Note: Pilates is designed with generally low rep schemes.

PILATES ADVANCED

Hundred

Roll ups

Roll over

Single leg circles

Single leg stretch

Double leg stretch

Single straight leg stretch

Double straight leg stretch

Crisscross

Open leg rocker

Corkscrew

Swan

Double leg kicks

Neck pull

Scissors

(continued on next page)

PILATES ADVANCED (Cont.)

Bicycle

Shoulder bridge

Spine twist

Jackknife

Side kicks

Teaser

Hip circles

Swimmers

Leg pulldown

Leg pull up

Kneeling side kicks

Mermaid

Boomerang

Seal

Pushup

Note: Pilates is designed with generally low rep schemes.

PILATES TYPES

Balanced Body

Basi

Classical

Contemporary

Fletcher Pilates

Jay Grimes

Lolita san Miguel

Mari Windsor

Peak

Romana

Stott

FITNESS TIP: Like every good fitness discipline, the individual must find the type that works best for them.

MAT PILATES ELEMENTS

Redefining the body

Your powerhouse

Scooping your belly

Tucking under vs. Lengthening

Integrated isolation

Stabilization using the pilates stance

Muscle control without tension

Modifications for the most common pains and injuries

Lengthening your neck

Reference: *The Pilates Body,* Brooke Siler, ©2000, Broadway Books, NY.

QIGONG BASIC

Raising the arms

Opening the chest

Paint a rainbow

Separate the clouds

Rolling the arms

Row a boat

Carry a ball in front

Gazing at the moon

Turning the waist

Cloud hands

Scooping the sea

Note: Qigong is designed for movement, breath and awareness. The Qigong wheel is a great finishing movement for aligning energy.

SUN SALUTATION A

Mountain pose, prayer

Mountain pose, raised arms

Forward fold pose

Half forward fold pose

High plank pose

Staff pose

Up dog pose

Down dog pose

Half forward fold pose

Forward fold pose

Mountain pose, hands overhead

Mountain pose, prayer

Note: Sun Salutations lengthens and strengthens, flexes and extends the main muscles of the body while creating a prana flow of energy throughout the system. http://yogapractice.tumblr.com

SUN SALUTATION B

Mountain pose

Chair pose

Forward fold pose

Half forward fold pose

High plank pose

Staff pose

Up dog pose

Down dog pose

Warrior I, right foot

High plank pose

Up dog pose

Down dog pose

Warrior I, left foot

High plank pose

Up dog pose

Down dog pose

Half forward fold pose

Forward fold pose

Chair pose

Mountain pose

Note: Sun Salutations lengthens and strengthens, flexes and extends the main muscles of the body while creating a prana flow of energy throughout the system. http://yogapractice.tumblr.com.

WOMEN'S HEALTH YOGA

nadi shodhana pranayama

surya namaskar A, use cobra not up dog

Childs pose

Cow pose

Lion pose

Butterfly pose

Reclined angle pose, pillow under hips

maha mudra

Revolved head to knee pose

Seated hero twist

Hero pose

Bridge pose, block under hips

Boat pose

Shoulder stand pose

Childs pose

Bow pose

Childs pose

Legs up wall pose

Childs pose

Note: Designed for women with distress of abdominal or hip region, internal or reproductive organs, neuromuscular or digestive issues. If menses present, do savasana with imagery at end of this pose sequence or healing meditation, and eliminate the shoulder stand pose.

YOGA BRANCHES

Jnana, self-inquiry, meditation and contemplation (Wisdom)

Bhakti, focuses on the Divine, or the heart.

Increasing tolerance, love, and acceptance of others (Devotion)

Karma, how our actions taken yesterday will affect our lives tomorrow and in the future

Raja, the act of meditation

Hatha, the act of performing what are called asanas (postures)

Tantra, rituals of yoga

Kriya, breathing techniques intended to purify and cleanse the body's energy channels

Kundalini, energy that lies dormant in the body until released

Mantra, words that are considered capable of creating transformation in yoga

YOGA TYPES

Ashtanga, a faster, more aerobic, flowing style of yoga

Bikram, hot Yoga developed by Bikram

Choudhury

Iyengar, known for its use of props, such as belts and blocks, as aids in performing postures

Jivamukti, incorporates ashtanga yoga with spiritual teachings and how to apply yogic philosophy to life

Kripalu, based on inner focus and meditation along with standard yoga poses and "breathwork," as well as "development of a quiet mind" and relaxation

Viniyoga, emphasizes the breath of yoga

Kundalini, releasing energy that lies in the body

Vinyasa, a style of yoga based on sequential postures and breathing (Flow)

Sivananda, five principles to develop physical, spiritual, and mental health

Forrest, focuses on breath, strength, integrity, and spirit

CHAPTER 5

Flexibility & Balance Workouts

FLEXIBILITY, including stretching training, refers to the absolute range of movement in a joint or series of joints, and length in muscles that cross the joints. Quality of life is enhanced by improving and maintaining a good range of motion in the joints. Overall flexibility should be developed with specific joint range of motion needs in mind as the individual joints vary from one to another. Loss of flexibility can be a predisposing factor for physical issues such as pain syndromes or balance disorders. (http://en.wikipedia.org)

BALANCE TRAINING. Static and dynamic exercises that are designed to improve individual's ability to withstand challenges from postural sway or destabilizing stimuli caused by self-motion, the environment, or other objects to improve balance, stability and function. (www.cdc.gov)

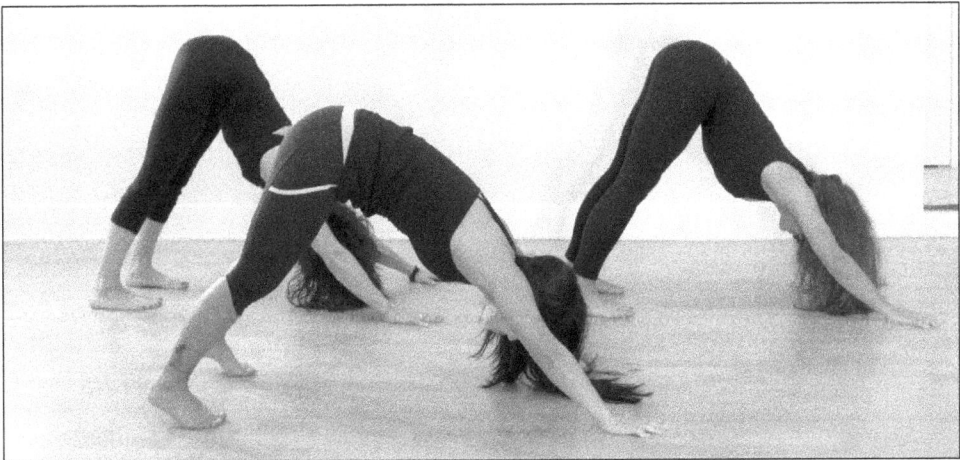

Downward dog

ABDOMINAL STRETCHES

Bar hang, toes drag behind on floor

Bow pose

Cat/dog

Cobra pose

Kneeling hands behind hips, hands on floor hip lift

Kneeling hands on hip back extension

Sphinx pose

Standing back extension

Supine arms overhead

Supine over stability ball

Note: For traditional static stretches to be effective, determine the correct muscle angle (function) and vary the stretch duration from 2–60 seconds.

BICEP STRETCHES

Arms straight overhead hands interlocked, palms up

Hands behind back lift

Hold barbell behind back, arms straight

Interlocked hands to front

Interlocked hands to overhead

Kneeling hands in front of knees, palms down, fingers pointed inward

One hand against wall twist, palm flat

One hand against wall twist, palm out

Seated hands on chair, palms down, fingers pointed back

Standing cross

Note: For traditional static stretches to be effective, determine the correct muscle angle (function) and vary the stretch duration from 2–60 seconds.

BODY WEIGHT BALANCE

1. One leg stand

2. One leg stand, eyes closed

3. One leg stand, on toes

4. One leg stand, on toes, eyes closed

5. Low plank, contralateral limbs elevated

6. High plank, contralateral limbs elevated

7. Reverse tabletop, contralateral limbs elevated

8. Boat pose or V sit isometric

9. Head stand (tripod)

10. Forearm stand

11. Hand stand

Note: Progress with eyes closed more often or use balance equipment such as a Bosu® ball.

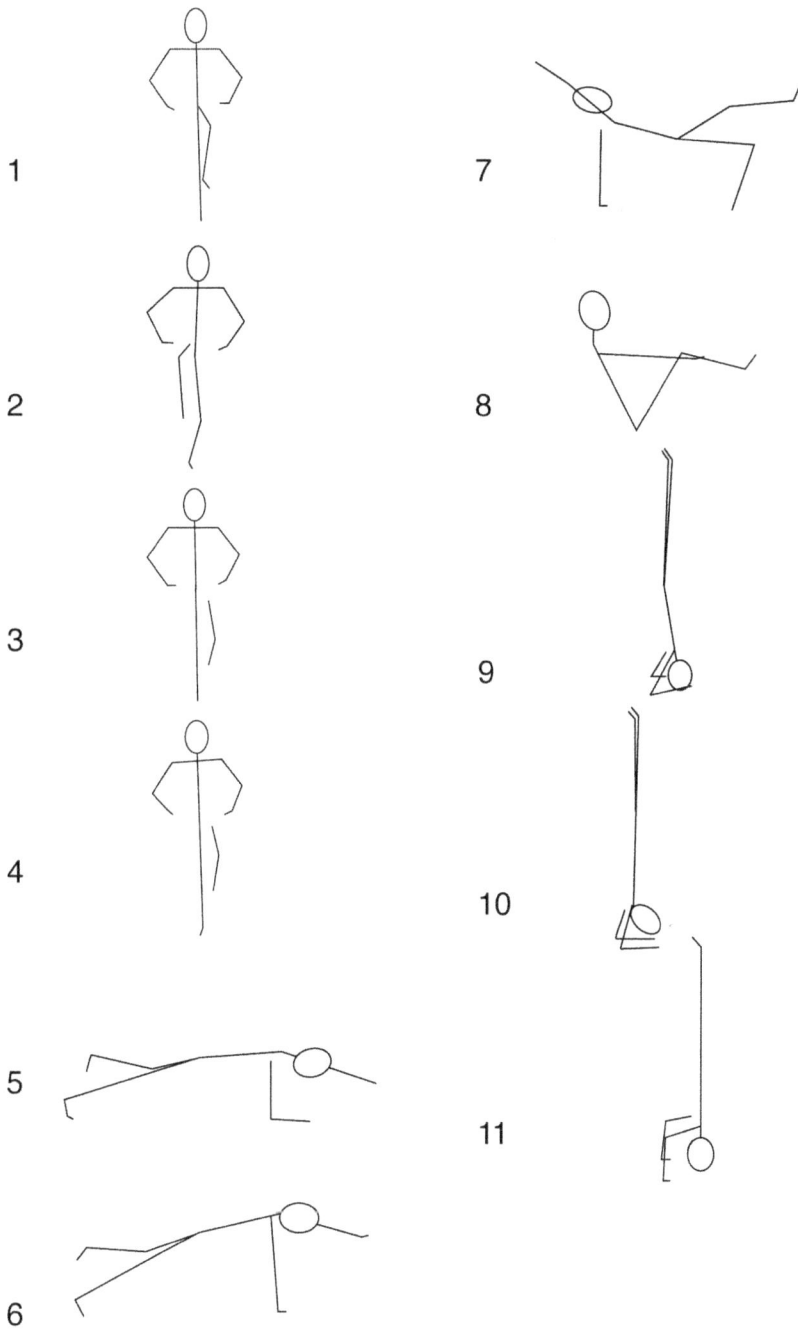

1

2

3

4

5

6

7

8

9

10

11

CALF STRETCHES

Bent knee foot inclined, hips forward

Bent knee foot inclined, hips forward hands on wall

Bent knee one leg heel drop on step

Bent knee standing split leg, back leg straight

Bent knee two leg heel drop on step

Foot inclined, hips forward

Foot inclined, hips forward hands on wall

One leg heel drop on step

Standing split leg, back leg straight

Two leg heel drop on step

Note: For traditional static stretches to be effective, determine the correct muscle angle (function) and vary the stretch duration from 2–60 seconds.

CERVICAL STRETCHES

Seated Extension

Seated flexion

Seated Retraction

Seated rotation

Seated Side bend

Supine extension

Supine retraction

Note: Perform 10 reps each exercise. Use the convex side or lean toward the convex area as directed. Based on McKenzie method.

CHEST & UPPER BACK STRETCHES

Bent over dumbbell hang to front, shoulder stretch

Myoball pressure chest area

Myoball pressure on anterior/lateral shoulder

Standing bent arm on wall, twist away from arm

Standing dumbbell hang to rear, shoulder stretch

Standing hands behind back, lift arms

Standing overhead shoulder stretch, hold strap overhead to feel shoulder stretch

Standing straight arm on wall, twist away from arm

Note: Perform 2–3 rounds, holding for approximately 30 seconds.

DELTOID STRETCHES

Arm arrest, one arm behind back, pull with other arm

Bent over straight arms on wall

Eagle prayer, interlocked forearms in front of chest

Interlocked forearms overhead

One arm across chest, other arm pushed inward on elbow

One arm against wall twist

One arm overhead, other arm behind back, grab fingers or towel

One arm overhead, pull elbow inward with other arm

Reverse prayer, behind back prayer

Supine over stability ball, arms out stretched

Note: For traditional static stretches to be effective, determine the correct muscle angle (function) and vary the stretch duration from 2–60 seconds.

FLEXIBILITY BASICS

As able, hold each successive stretch deeper and exhale as increasing stretch

Consider PNF stretching

Determine function of tight muscle, at getbodysmart.com. From this, a proper stretch can be utilized.

Find the correct angle of the stretch which should actually lengthen the muscle

Hold each stretch for 30 seconds, do 2–3 sets per stretch

Stretch all muscles/groups unless contraindicated

Stretch between weight training sets

Stretch for functionality or sport specificity

Stretch when warmed up and relax when stretching

Use a variety of stretches

Note: The "Sun Salutation" is one of the most complete and effective functional flexibility routines.

FOREARM STRETCHES

Interlocked hands behind back

Interlocked hands overhead

Interlocked hands to front

Kneeling fingers backward lean back

Kneeling fingers forward lean forward

Prayer, hand to hand

Spider hold, straight arm forward, fingers spread

Straight arm, fingers down, pull fingers back

Straight arm, fingers up, pull fingers back

Wrist rotations

Note: For traditional static stretches to be effective, determine the correct muscle angle (function) and vary the stretch duration from 2–60 seconds.

FULL BODY STRETCHES

Extended childs pose

Forward fold

Frog pose

Kneeling, Japanese seated position

Mountain, arms overhead

Seated counter stretch

Seated spinal twist

Seated wide leg forward fold

Standing back extension

Standing cross stretch, for biceps

Supine double knee in

Supine hamstring stretch

Supine single knee in

Supine spinal twist

Supine straight leg across body

Supine straight leg lateral

Note: Perform one round of 20–40 seconds. Repeat any as needed 1–2 more times

GLUTE STRETCHES

Myoroller glute sit

Medicine ball (or myoball) glute sit

Seated cross leg, knee push down

Seated one leg bent knee pull

Sprinter, face down forward split

Supine cross leg pull in

Supine one ankle on knee pull

Supine one leg bent knee pull

Supine one leg bent knee twist

Supine two leg bent knee pull

Note: For traditional static stretches to be effective, determine the correct muscle angle (function) and vary the stretch duration from 2–60 seconds.

HAMSTRING STRETCHES

Seated one leg straight, other foot to thigh forward bend

Seated straight leg forward bend

Standing cross leg, forward bend

Standing leg on bench forward bend

Standing toe touch

Supine one leg bent, other leg straight on wall

Supine one leg slightly bent knee pull in

Supine one leg straight knee pull in, other leg bent

Supine one leg straight knee pull in, other leg straight

Supine two leg slightly bent knees pull in

Note: For traditional static stretches to be effective, determine the correct muscle angle (function) and vary the stretch duration from 2–60 seconds.

HIP ABDUCTOR STRETCHES

Single knee twist pull

Standing cross leg, 45° bend

Standing cross leg, one arm on wall lean

Standing cross leg, side bend

Standing split stance, side bend

Supine bent knee twist

Supine cross leg pull

Supine single cross leg, one leg straight on floor, other leg straight across body

Supine single knee twist, knee over other leg

Note: These stretches are also great for the Iliotibial band, the fascial layer that runs down the outside of the leg from the hip to knee.

HIP ADDUCTOR STRETCHES

Frog, seated wide leg straight leg toes hold

Leg adductor machine flex

One leg on chair, other on floor, forward bend

Prone frog pose

Seated butterfly forward bend

Seated or supine butterfly

Seated wide leg forward bend

Seated wide straight legs, feet against wall

Side lunge, standing side squat, one leg straight, one leg bent

Sumo squat

Note: For traditional static stretches to be effective, determine the correct muscle angle (function) and vary the stretch duration from 2–60 seconds.

HIP STRETCHES WITH STRAP

Supine single knee to chest

Supine straight leg to chest

Supine straight leg to chest with strap

Supine straight leg to side, abduction with strap

Supine straight leg to side, adduction with strap

Spinal twist

Note: Repeat other leg. Do 2–3 rounds of 20–40 seconds per stretch.

LAT STRETCHES

Extended childs pose

Hanging from bar

Kneeling straight arm on stability ball

Prayer, kneeling, head and straight arms on ground

Pulling on overhead post

Seated bent knee thigh grab

Seated cross leg forward bend, arms outstretched

Standing bent over pull on bar

Supine knee in rolls

Supine over medicine ball

Note: For traditional static stretches to be effective, determine the correct muscle angle (function) and vary the stretch duration from 2–60 seconds.

LUMBAR STRETCHES

Cat/dog

Childs pose

Cobra pose

Seated bent knee toe touch

Seated straight leg forward bend

Sphinx pose

Standing cross leg toe touch

Standing toe touch

Supine one leg bent knee pull in

Supine over stability ball

Supine two leg bent knee pull in

Note: For traditional static stretches to be effective, determine the correct muscle angle (function) and vary the stretch duration from 2–60 seconds.

MYOCORE WORKOUT UPPER BODY

Anterior deltoid, prone myoball under shoulder, roll around front of shoulder

Chest, prone myoball under chest, roll around front of chest

Ab, prone, ball under abs, gently roll around abdominal area, use caution

Supine neck, ball under neck to one side, roll back and forth around neck

Supine traps, ball under shoulders, roll around trap area

Supine lats, ball under shoulders, roll around lat area

Supine mid back, ball under mid back, roll around mid-back area

Seated glute, ball under glute, roll around hip area

Prone hip flexor, ball under front hip, roll around hip area

Note: This is a core class with the use of a myoball. Avoid direct pressure on spine with ball.

MYOCORE WORKOUT LOWER BODY

Hamstrings, seated on myoroller, hands on floor, roll back and forth on both hamstrings

Calves, seated on myoroller, hands on floor, roll back and forth on both calves

Single hamstring, seated on myoroller, hands on floor, roll back and forth on hamstring, switch

Single calf, seated on myoroller, hands on floor, roll back and forth on calf, switch

Outer thigh, myoroller under outer thigh, top leg foot on floor, roll back and forth on outer thigh

Inner thigh, myoroller under inner thigh, roll back and forth on inner thigh

Outer thigh, myoroller under outer thigh, top leg parallel to bottom leg, roll over outer thigh

Lumbar, seated with myoroller on low back, roll up and down on low back area

Note: This is a core class with the use of a myoroller. Avoid direct pressure on spine with myoroller.

MULTI-MUSCLE STRETCHES

Cobra pose

Down dog pose

Extended childs pose

Low lunge pose

Mountain pose, hands raised

Prone over stability ball

Standing forward fold pose

Supine bent knee torso twist

Supine over stability ball

Triangle pose

Up dog pose

Warrior pose

Note: For traditional static stretches to be effective, determine the correct muscle angle (function) and vary the stretch duration from 2–60 seconds.

OBLIQUE STRETCHES

Kneeling side bend

Seated arms behind head torso twist

Seated bar twist

Seated yoga twist

Side over hyper extension machine

Side over stability ball

Standing bar twist

Standing side bend

Supine bent knee twist

Supine straight leg twist

Note: For traditional static stretches to be effective, determine the correct muscle angle (function) and vary the stretch duration from 2–60 seconds.

PECTORAL STRETCHES

Arms on door jam forward lean

Bent over straight arms on wall twist

One arm against wall twist

Seated hands behind neck, back extension

Standing hands on glutes, push elbows back

Supine arms overhead

Supine over medicine ball

Supine over stability ball, arms out stretched

Towel straight arm overhead

Note: For traditional static stretches to be effective, determine the correct muscle angle (function) and vary the stretch duration from 2–60 seconds.

QUADRICEP STRETCHES

Bow pose

Childs Pose

Kneeling one leg forward, hands on knee

One foot on high bench, dip down

Prone knee bend

Prone lower thigh on foam knee bend

Prone one bent knee, other leg straight

Runner's stretch

Side lying knee bend

Standing knee bend

Note: These stretches may also target the Hip flexors.

TRAPEZIUS STRETCHES

Bent over straight arms on wall

One arm across chest, other arm pushed inward on elbow

One arm against wall twist

One arm overhead, other arm behind back, grab fingers or towel

One arm overhead, pull elbow inward with other arm

Prayer, interlocked forearms in front of chest

Reverse prayer, behind back prayer

Supine arms overhead

Supine over stability ball, arms out stretched

Towel straight arm overhead

Note: For traditional static stretches to be effective, determine the correct muscle angle (function) and vary the stretch duration from 2–60 seconds.

TRICEP STRETCHES

Arms elbows behind neck

Interlocked hands to overhead

Interlocked hands, one behind neck, other behind mid back

Kneeling elbows bent overhead on chair, lean down

Overhead bent elbow stretch, hand by neck

Overhead bent elbow stretch, hand by neck, pull elbow in

Overhead bent elbow stretch, hand by shoulder

Overhead bent elbow stretch, hand by shoulder, pull elbow in

Staff pose, position with hands on floor, elbows up

Towel stretch, one behind neck, other behind mid back

Note: For traditional static stretches to be effective, determine the correct muscle angle (function) and vary the stretch duration from 2–60 seconds.

MYOROLLER WORKOUT LOWER BODY

Hamstring (sit with myoroller below thigh)

Calf (sit with myoroller below calf)

Quad (prone with myoroller below thigh)

Outer thigh (lie sideways with myoroller under thigh)

Inner thigh (prone with myoroller under inner thigh)

Gluteals (sit on myoroller under glutes)

Shin (kneel with myoroller under shins)

Ankles (roll myoroller on all sides of ankle)

Feet (roll myoroller on tops of feet with hands)

FITNESS TIP: We cannot underestimate the importance of foot health.

MYOROLLER WORKOUT UPPER BODY

Low back (Supine with myoroller under low back, caution required)

Obliques (Lie sideways with myoroller under side below ribs)

Abs (Prone, roll myoroller on abs gently with arms, caution required)

Bolster for chest and back (Supine with myoroller under mid back between shoulder blades)

Lats (Lie sideways with myoroller under arms/shoulder blade)

Triceps (sideways with myoroller under triceps)

Biceps (prone with myoroller under biceps)

Shoulder (kneeling with myoroller under arm on bench or chair)

Neck (supine with myoroller under cervicals, caution required)

YOGA BALANCE

1. Triangle pose

2. High lunge pose

3. Half moon pose

4. Hand to big toe pose

5. Tree pose

6. Warrior I pose

7. Warrior II pose

8. Warrior III pose

9. Eagle pose

10. Lord of the dance pose

11. Crow pose

12. Crane pose

Note: For progression, perform with one or both eyes closed

1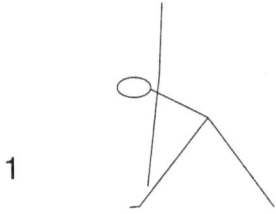

7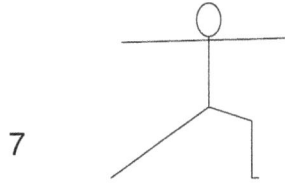

2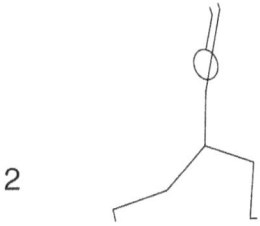

8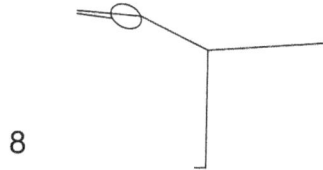

3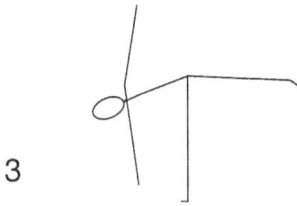

9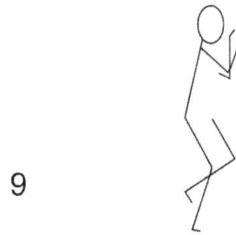

4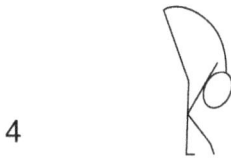

11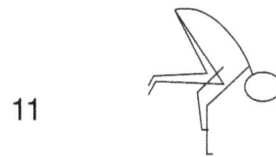

5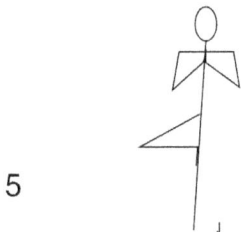

12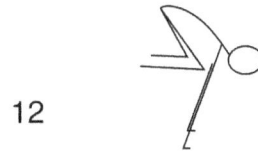

6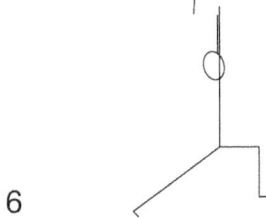

STABILITY BALL BALANCE BASIC

Standing two leg

Standing two leg, one eye closed

Standing two leg, eyes closed

Kneeling with toes elevated

Kneeling with toes elevated eyes closed

Seated one foot elevated

Seated both feet elevated

Seated both feet elevated eyes closed

Superman, torso on ball, limbs elevated

One leg hip lift, head/shoulders on ball

One leg low plank, forearms on ball

Note: Caution, only attempt if confident of results. Progression can include adding Chop, Twist, Arm raise, Leg raise, Squat, Eye(s) closed, etc. For progression, add movement and/or weight resistance.

STABILITY BALL BALANCE INTERMEDIATE

Chair (seated on ball, feet off floor)

Boat (seated on ball with heels close to glutes, feet off floor)

Jockey (seated on ball with knees wide, feet off floor)

Four point knees (hands and knees on ball)

Four point feet (hands and feet on ball)

Four point forearms (forearms and knees on ball)

Three point (one hand and knees on ball)

Two point (both knees on ball)

Two point (one hand, one knee on ball)

One point balance (Superman on ball)

FITNESS TIP: Proper core stability and activation leads to progress in all other areas of fitness.

STABILITY BALL BALANCE ADVANCED

1. Seated chair

2. Seated boat

3. Seated jockey

4. Four point hands/knees

5. Four point hands/feet

6. Four point forearms/knees

7. Four point forearms/feet

8. Four point reverse table pose

9. Three point hands/one arm up

10. Three point hands/one knee up

11. Three point hands/feet arm up

12. Three point hands/feet leg up

13. Three point forearm/knees arm up

14. Three point forearm/knees up

15. Three point forearm/feet arm up

16. Three point forearm/feet leg up

17. Three point reverse table pose

18. Two point knees

19. Two point standing

20. Two point one arm/one knee

21. Two point one forearm/one knee

Note: Caution, only attempt if confident of results

1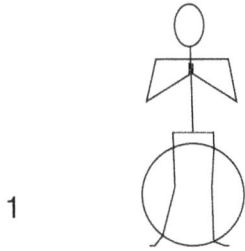

2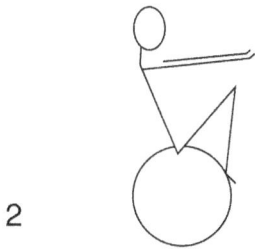

3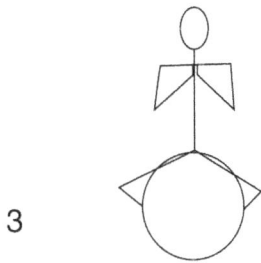

4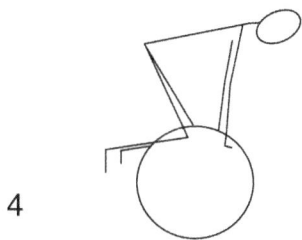

5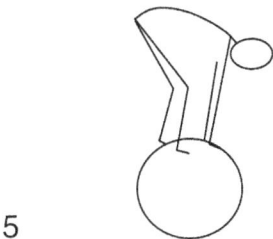

6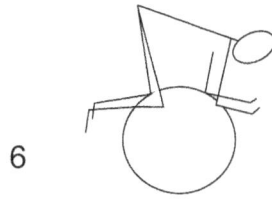

7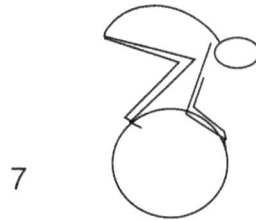

8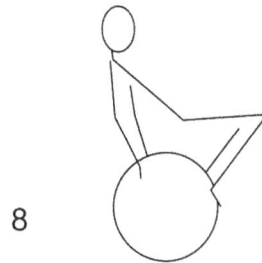

9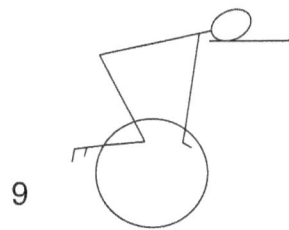

10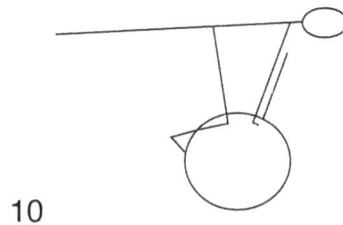

11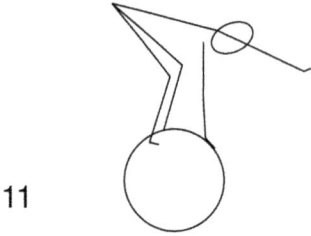

16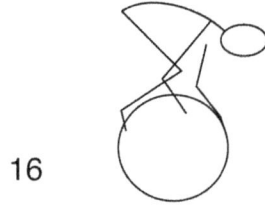

12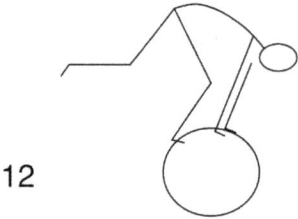

18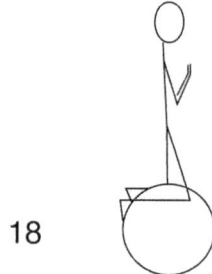

13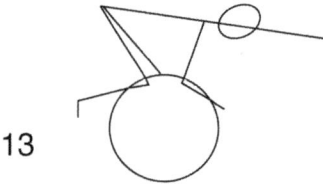

19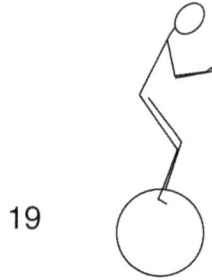

14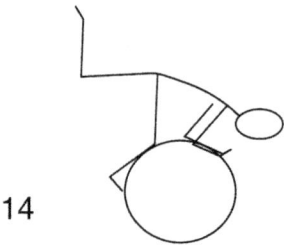

20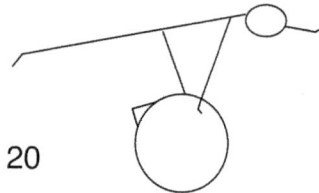

15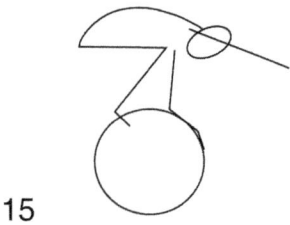

21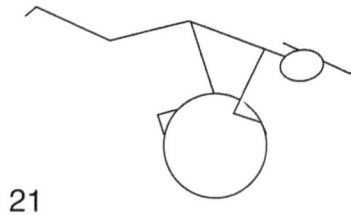

MASSAGE TYPES

Aromatherapy, therapeutic use of aromatic plant extracts and essential oils

Ayurveda and yoga

Deep tissue, designed to relieve severe tension in the muscle and the connective tissue or fascia

Myofascial release, technique for stretching the fascia and releasing bonds between fascia, integument, and muscles

Reiki, technique of transmitting life energy by placing the hands gently in specific positions either on or above the body

Shiatsu, applied pressure with thumbs, fingers, and palms to the same energy meridians as acupressure, uses stretching

Sports, designed to enhance athletic performance and recovery

Stone Therapy, uses cold or water-heated stones to apply pressure and heat to the body

Swedish, uses five styles of long, flowing strokes to massage

Thai, originated in India and is based on

Therapeutic, involves acting on and manipulating the body with pressure

CHAPTER 6

Virtual Workouts & Online Fitness

VIRTUAL WORKOUTS are some of the favorite workouts the author has used periodically for his virtual clientele. There is a break after every series or full set (numbered sections, 1, 2, 3, etc.) unless otherwise noted. For unilaterally exercises like lunges or side planks, 20 reps means 10 reps each side. Additional rest periods may be noted.

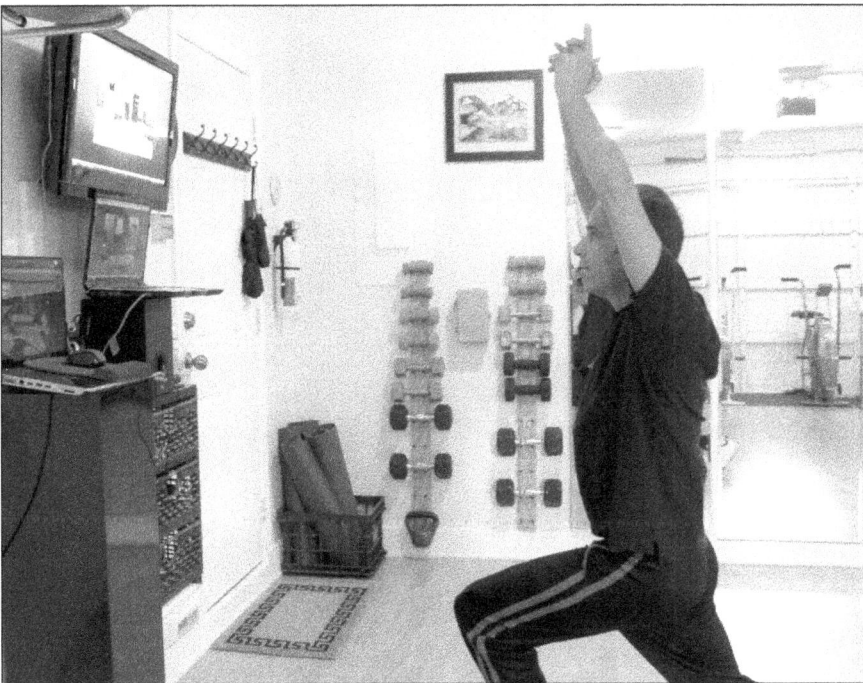

Virtual training

VIRTUAL TRAINING SAMPLE SERIES

The following VPT workouts are based on this basic outline of reps and sets.

Example One:

Lunge

Squat

Crunch – 3x30 seconds, repeat 3 times

Participant does the three exercises in a row, each one for 30 seconds, then repeat the whole 3 times total, taking a break between each of the three sets.

Example Two:

Burpees – 1x8

Participant does do the one exercise 8 reps/times, just one time.

Example Three:

Pushup

Pull up

Situp – 3x20, 3x15, 3x12, no break

Participant does the 3 exercises in a row, 20 times each, then all 3 in a row 15 times each.

BURPEE HEAVEN VPT WORKOUT

Burpees – 1x5

Crunches

Jump squat – 3x30 seconds, repeat 3 times

Burpees – 1x10

Medicine ball chop – 1x20

Burpees – 1x15

Situp

Crunch – 2x12

Burpees – 1x20

One leg deadlift – 1x20

Burpees – 1x15

Superman

Pushup – 2x20, 2x15, 2x12

Burpees – 1x10

Squat

Lunge – 2x20, 3x15, 3x12

Burpees – 1x5

Plank – 1x1 minute

Burpees – 1x25

FITNESS TIP: Learn proper form and the various types and techniques of burpees and squat thrusts.

BURPEES & CORE VPT WORKOUT

Crunches – 1x15

Burpees – 1x8

Corkscrew

Side crunch

Medicine ball chop – 3x20, 3x15, 3x12

Burpees – 1x10

Situp

Reverse crunch

Crunch – 3x20, 3x15, 3x12

Burpees – 1x12, rest, 1x15, rest, 1x20

Squat twist

Lunge twist – 2x20, 2x15, 2x12

Burpees – 1x25

Note: Focus on using your core muscles for all movements and stabilizations.

CARDIO TWISTER VPT WORKOUT

Jump rope turning 90 degrees each jump – 3x30 seconds

Crunch with twist

Lunge with twist

Wide grip pull ups with leg twist – 3x20

Situp with twist

Deadlift with lifting twist

Tricep dip – 3x20

Crunch with twist

Two leg calf raise with dumbbell

Curl grip pull up with leg twist – 3x20

Corkscrew

Romanian deadlift

Cable cross chest fly – 3x20

(continued on next page)

CARDIO TWISTER VPT WORKOUT (Cont.)

Lunge with twist

Squat with twist

Mason twist

Scorpion

Santana pushup – 5x20,

Jumping jacks

Low jack

Jump rope

Jumping jacks – 4x90 seconds

Note: Repeat entire workout 1–6.

FITNESS TIP: For stretching and rehab purposes, it is recommended to have myoball, baseball, myoroller, golf ball, softball and yoga strap/belt

CRAZY CARDIO CIRCUIT VPT WORKOUT

Stair running (jog in place), 2 minutes

Crunch

Reverse crunch

Bench reverse crunch

V situp

Teaser

Wood chop – 6x30

Corkscrew

Side plank hip lift

V situp

Stability ball roll out – 4x25

Lunge

Jump lunge

Traveling lunge – 3x25

(continued on next page)

CRAZY CARDIO CIRCUIT VPT WORKOUT (Cont.)

Superman

Birddog

Lunge and reach – 3x20

Squat

Lunge

Leg press or back lunge

Leg extension or one leg lunge

Traveling lunge – 5x20

Note: Attempt no breaks until the end; rinse and repeat!

CORE CRUSHER VPT WORKOUT

Burpees – 1x20

Corkscrew – 1x20

Teaser

Side plank hip lift – 2x20

Stability ball bridge

Stability ball back extension

Crunch legs on stability ball – 3x20

Stability ball walkout

Ab roller roll out

Medicine ball chop

Medicine ball crunch – 4x20

Crisscross

Twist situp

Stability ball walkout

Mason twist – 4x40

Burpees – 1x20

Note: Focus on using your core muscles for all movements and stabilizations.

DO IT ALL! VPT WORKOUT

Crunch

Situp

V situp

Crunch – 4x20, repeat 2 times, no break

One leg calf raise

Squat – 2x30, 2x24, 2x20

Pushup plank – 1x90 seconds

Pull up or bent over row

Superman

Low side plank hip lift

Cable cross over chest fly – 4x20, rest, 4x15, rest, 4x12

Tricep dip

Close grip pushup – 2x20, repeat 3 times, no break

Pushup plank – 1x90 seconds

V situp

Crunch

V situp – 3x20, repeat 3 times, no break

Forearm plank, one leg up – 1x2 minutes

Leg press, moderate weight, or squat – 1x100 (not a typo)

Note: Focus on good form and integration to use all muscles functionally.

FULL BODY BLITZ VPT WORKOUT

Alternate toe touch

Burpees

Jump squat – 3x1 minute

Crunch/Situp/Crunch – 3x20, repeat 3 times, no break

V situp/Situp/V situp – 3x20, repeat 3 times

One leg calf raise

Squat – 2x30, 2x24, 2x20

One leg calf raise

Lunge – 2x30, 2x24, 2x20, no break

Pull up/Superman/Side low plank hip lift

Pushup – 4x20, rest, 4x15, rest, 4x12

Tricep dip

Close grip pushup – 2x20, repeat 3 times

Crunch/Reverse crunch/Crunch – 3x20, repeat 3 times, no break

Up dog/down

High/low plank

Teaser/V situp – 3x20, repeat 3 times, no break

FITNESS TIP: Teasers and V-up done in pilates fashion are an excellent core exercise.

GET UP! VPT WORKOUT

Get ups – 1x5

Alternate toe touch

Burpees

Jumping jacks – 3x30 seconds, repeat 3 times

Get ups – 1x8

Corkscrew

Side plank isometric

Pull up or bent over row – 3x20, 3x15, 3x12

Get ups – 1x10

Situp

Reverse crunch

Tricep dip – 3x20, 3x15, 3x12

Get ups – 1x12

Birddog

One leg deadlift

Dumbbell bicep curl – 3x20, 3x15, 3x12

Burpees – 1x15

Side lying hip lift

Superman

Pushups – 3x20, 3x15, 3x12

Burpees – 1x20

FITNESS TIP: Take half your weight, that's how many ounces of water is recommended per day.

HUNDREDS VPT WORKOUT

Get ups – 1x5

Situp – 1x100

Bicep curl – 1x100

Calf raise – 1x100

Teaser – 1x100

Overhead dumbbell press – 1x100

Light dumbbell deadlift – 1x100

Traveling side squat – 1x100

Pushup – 1x50

Tricep dip – 1x100

Superman – 1x100

Pull up – 1x50

Burpees – 1x20

Note: Take as few breaks as possible to get to 50 or 100 reps

UNILATERAL VPT WORKOUT

Forearm plank, one leg suspended – 1x90 seconds

Crunch/Situp/Crunch– 3x20, repeat 3x

Forearm plank, one leg suspended – 1x90 seconds

One leg calf raise

Squat – 2x30, 2x24, 2x20

One leg calf raise

Lunge – 2x30, 2x24, 2x20

Forearm plank, one leg suspended – 1x90 seconds

Pull up/Superman

Side low plank hip lift

Pushup, one leg suspended – 4x20, rest, 4x15, rest, 4x12

Forearm plank, one leg suspended – 1x90 seconds

Crunch one leg suspended

Crunch one leg suspended – 2x20, repeat 3x

> **FITNESS TIP:** Add Up dog/down, One leg suspended, One leg bicep curl, One leg overhead press, One leg tricep extension, One leg bent over row – 5x20, repeat 2x.

WALKING THE PLANK VPT WORKOUT

High/low plank – 1x90 seconds

Crunch

Situp

V situp

Crunch – 4x20, repeat 2 times, no break

High/low plank – 1x90 seconds

One leg calf raise

Squat – 2x30, 2x24, 2x20

High/low plank – 1x90 seconds

Pull up

Superman

Low side plank hip lift

Cable cross over chest fly – 4x20, rest, 4x15, rest, 4x12

High/low plank – 1x90 seconds

Crunch

Reverse crunch

Accordion crunch – 3x20, repeat 3 times, no break

High/low plank – 1x90 seconds

QUALIFIED VPT ATTRIBUTES

Adaptable, must be flexible to give client proper, well-rounded wellness

Articulate, must have good verbal non-demonstrative directives

Attentive, must situate client properly to be able to view form and function and stays focused on client throughout session

Certified and qualified

Computer skills, must understand basic skype, pc and Mac hardware and software

Have a well-lit, comfortable area for both trainer and client

Participates in online sessions themselves and well as other recorded video classes

Punctual, must call client on time

Work with the client individually, even if a group setting

RECOMMENDATIONS FOR VPT CLIENTS

Carpet, mat or towel

Computer or smart phone w/camera

Desire to be well

Empty wall or door space (about 2 feet wide)

Sturdy kitchen chair

Teleconferencing software installed (eg, Skype, Hangout)

Water

FITNESS TIP: Some optional but helpful equipment for the trainee includes a 65cm Stability ball, Exercise/yoga mat, Theraband, Bosu ball, Dumbbells and Iron Gym

SMART PHONE FITNESS APPS

C25K

Fitness Builder

GoodFoodNearYou

GymGoal ABC

iFitness

iTreadmill

Lose it

Men's Fitness

Nutrition Tips

RunKeeper Pro

Reference: Best Fitness Apps, Got an iPhone? Then it's time to stop texting and start flexing , Lisa Freedman, www.mensfitness.com/ training/best-fitness-apps, June 2012.

TOP VPT CLASSES

Demandfitness.com

Physii.com

Virtualgym.tv/index.aspx

VirtualPersonalTrainers.net

Virtucise.net

VirtuFit.net

Yogaglo.com

Yogalearningcenter.com

FITNESS TIP: Check out ideafit.com for great health and fitness tips.

VIRTUAL GYM ESSENTIALS

Balance disks

Bike or treadmill

Body bars®

Bosu Ball

Cybex Multi-station

Dumbbells

Exercise bands

FreeMotion® Cable Cross

Medicine balls

Power blocks®

Stability ball

Workout bench

FITNESS TIP: Cable machines offering a great range of exercises; be creative and safe and experiment with good form to find new movements to strengthen the body.

VPT COURSE OUTLINE

The VPT certification process takes about 4 weeks following basic program outline. Each is detailed on the following pages.

Skype/Facetime

Office Setup

Virtual Equipment

Fitness Equipment

Fitness Fees

Virtual Routines

Virtual Group exercise

Client relations

Fitness Website

General Marketing

e-Marketing

Education

VPT LEVEL I

The VPT must meet the following requirements before becoming certified.

Age 18 or older

Certification (eg, Pilates, Yoga, cycling)

Creativity and open-mindedness with a passion for wellness

Current CPR Certification

Current Personal Trainer or Group Exercise

Device w/camera

Teleconferencing software (eg, Skype)

This manual

FITNESS TIP: Focus on the health you have and would like to continue and improve. Steer free of negative thoughts about your health.

VPT LEVEL II

Those requirements for VPT I

Train 50 or more webcam client hours

Listed on /www.virtualpersonaltrainers.net

Develop website dedicated to your VPT business

Read VPT manual 1st edition www.createspace.com/4428594

Read VPT manual 2nd Edition

FITNESS TIP: Take one day off training per week for recovery.

VPT CRITIQUE CRITERIA

Articulation (Word choice)

Audio quality

Communication (Client connection, my day)

Cooldown

Distraction (Background, noises)

Energy (Body language)

Exercise choice

Professionalism (Promptness, etc.)

Safety (Injuries, etc.)

Understanding (Speed of Speech)

Video quality

Warmup

FITNESS TIP: The two keys to Webcam training is the client *hearing* the trainer and the trainer *seeing* the client.

VPT 1 SKYPE/FACETIME

Audio quality

Close all programs

Connection speed

Mac/pc compatibility

Multipoint

Oovoo, facetime, hangout, etc.

Say hello

Seem them, hear you

Share screen

Skype icons (mike, add, video, etc.)

Skype IM

Video quality

VPT 2 OFFICE SETUP

Address/emergency

Aware of camera angle

Background

Background noise

Client's room

Device high, tilted down

Lighting

Mirror

Noise is amplified

Prop iPad

Safety

Space

Stand, sit on ball

Table, counter

Trainer's appearance

Trainer's room

Wear footware

VPT 3 VIRTUAL SETUP

Headset

Initial set up session with client

Keep phone on mute

Large TV

Smart Phone backup

Speakers

Use 2 or more devices simultaneously

Wired keyboard

VPT 4 FITNESS EQUIPMENT

Basic equipment

Belt/Strap

Chair

Counter

Has a gym

Iron gym

Laundry detergent, cans, etc.

Mat/Towel

Myoball, myorollers, etc.

Peak pilates

Perform better

Power systems

Proper footware

Stairs

Table

Wall

VPT 5 FITNESS FEES

Discounts

How much

Monthly fee

Paypal

Sending invoices

Session packages

Square, Paypal for credit cards

Upcharge (Credit cards, Debit cards, etc.)

VPT 6 VIRTUAL ROUTINES

Cardio

Core

Creativity

Flex

Groups

Importance of Stability ball

Individual

Intuition

Isometric

Keep routine notebook

Pilates

Recommended books (VPTM, FBL, etc.)

Strength

Variety

Yoga

VPT 7 VIRTUAL GROUP EXERCISE

Brain gym

Client relations

Duets, trios

Homework

Income via group sessions

Multiple devices

Multipoint

Nutrition, mental, cognitive, etc.

PT software

Punctuality

Studio & skype workouts together

Yoga, bootcamp, etc.

VPT 8 CLIENT RELATIONS

Brief

Clear

Client energy

Client volume

Client's mentality

Cues

Email support

Intuition

Non-demonstrative

Stand away from device

Text client for prep

Text support

Use of cc:, bcc:

What have they done

VPT 9 FITNESS WEBSITE

Email

Fees

Health Questionnaire

Key words

Meta tags

PR

SEO

Testimonials

Videos

VPT 10 VPT GENERAL MARKETING

50% discount for referral

Complimentary session

Current clientele

Email, text, etc.

Ideafit, AFAA, etc.

Newsletter Monthly

Presentations

Skype, Google+, etc.

Specials

Teach community class

VPT 11 VPT e-MARKETING

Facebook Ad

Facebook, Personal & Fan

GoDaddy, Wix, etc

Google ad

Marketing, Social Media

Metatags, keywords, etc.

SEO

Twitter, LinkedIn, Myspace, etc.

Visibility

VPT 12 FITNESS EDUCATION

Business Certifications

CEUs, CECs

Classes

Other fitness Certifications

Workshops

FITNESS TIP: A qualified VPT will listen and observe, talk minimally but directly, being ever vigilant.

CHAPTER 7

General Fitness & Safety

FITNESS is the state or condition of being fit; suitability or appropriateness; Good health or physical condition, especially as the result of exercise and proper nutrition. (www.thefreedictionary.com/fitness)

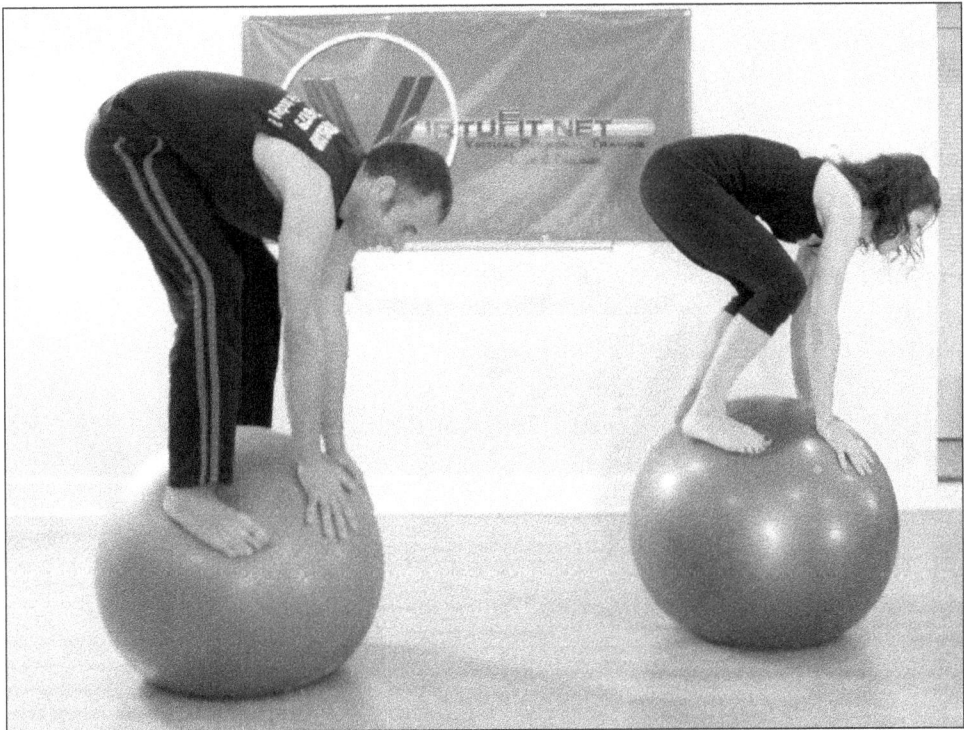

Stability ball exercise

12 MYTHS OR MISUNDERSTANDINGS

The first key to health is a positive attitude

The second key is consuming an organic GMO-free variety of healthy whole foods

The third key to health is regular meditation and proper recovery (see Chapter 3)

Train posterior muscles 2:1 over anterior

There are times when a knee can ride past an ankle in squat and lunge movements

Sometimes one needs to eat *more* to lose weight

Weight scales, for all intents and purposes, are useless

SMR with myoball and myoroller are more effective than traditional static stretching

DOMS is not good or bad, it merely means trainee performed something either new or excessive

A sore low back after a workout is usually good

More is not better, *better* is better

You should not separate mind, body and spirit from fitness

20–30'S FITNESS

Cardiovascular training

Challenge yourself

Core training

Free Weight Training

Lay groundwork for later in life

Low Reps

Play sports such as running, golf, biking, or tennis

Plyometric training

Speed-Agility-Quickness training

Strength training

Team sports

Reference: "Fitness Plans for the Ages," *Palm Beach Post*, Sunday, November 27, 2005.

40–50'S FITNESS

Balance training

Cardiovascular training

Core training

Flexibility training

Keep boredom at bay

Mental training

Play sports such as tennis, golf

Strength training

Vary activities

Reference: "Fitness Plans for the Ages," *Palm Beach Post*, Sunday, November 27, 2005

60–70'S FITNESS

Cardiovascular training

Core/Balance training

Functional training

Get proper Rest

Keep it real, exercise appropriately for age

Mental training

Pay attention to your body

Play sports as able, e.g., golf

Strength training

Tai Chi/Aquatics

Reference: "Fitness Plans for the Ages," *Palm Beach Post*, Sunday, November 27, 2005

AVOIDING WEIGHT ROOM INJURY

Be aware of your surroundings

Before you execute a lift, ensure all of the weight plates are secured

If training alone, be very aware of your capabilities and surroundings

If training outdoors, try to train in the morning during hot months

Practice perfect form

Stop exercising if you feel dizzy or like fainting

Use a safe lifting speed and avoid using momentum

Warm up before you move on to heavier weights

Wear appropriate workout clothing

When in doubt, ask for help

Reference: "Top 10 Tips to Get the Most Out of Your Bodybuilding Program . . . Safely," Hugo Rivera, About.com Guide, http://bodybuilding.about.com/od/injurypreventiontreatment /tp/trainingsafe.htm, June 2012

COMMON WEIGHT LIFTING INJURIES

Back Sprains and Strains

Herniated Disk

Patellar Tendinitis

Rotator Cuff Tear

Shoulder Impingement Syndrome

FITNESS TIP: Always be sure to stretch your muscles well before you lift weights. Making sure that your muscles are warmed up before your workout begins is a great way to avoid strains, sprains, tears and other common weight lifting injuries. Reduce your swelling by taking anti-inflammatory medications. You can also take supplements or eat foods high in omega-3 fatty acids, as these are known to help with inflammation. You can also apply ice packs sparingly to help reduce swelling. Often, weight lifters make the problem worse by continuing to do these exercises even when they begin to feel pain. One of the best steps for weight lifters in preventing injuries is to be aware of their body.

Reference: "Most Common Weight Lifting Injuries and How to Treat Them," Ashley Henshaw, September 15, 2011, www.symptomfind.com/ healthy-living/common-weight-lifting-injuries, June 2012

COMMON INJURIES

Ankle

Elbow

Hip

Knee

Lower back

Neck

Shoulder

Wrist

Note: For more information on the movements of the particular sport and designing strengthening and injury prevention training programs, go to csathleticdevelopment.co.uk/2.html.

COMMON RUNNERS INJURIES

Achilles tendinitis

Ankle sprains

Blisters

Dizziness/Nausea

Iliotibial band syndrome

Muscle pulls

Plantar fasciitis

Runner's knee

Shin splints

Stress fractures

Reference: WedMD, aolsvhealth.webmd.aol.com/content/article/61/67443.htm, June 2005

COMMON SPORTS INJURIES

Muscle pull

Achilles tendinitis

Ankle sprain

Foot Arch pain/strain

Lower back strain

Neck strain/pain

Runner's Knee

Shin splints

Shoulder impingement

Tennis Elbow

Reference: Cell Health Makeover, cellhealthmakeover.com/mostcommon-sports-injuries.html, June 2005; Sports Injury Handbooks, sportsinjuryhandbook.com/injuries, June 2005.

CERTIFICATION ORGANIZATIONS

AAAI/ISMA, New Hope, PA, 609-397-2139

Aerobics and Fitness Associations of America, Sherman Oaks, CA
877-968-7263

American College of Sports Medicine • 317-637-9200

American Council on Exercise, San Diego, CA,
800–825–3636

International Fitness Professionals Association, Tampa, FL
800-785-1924

National Exercise Trainers Association • 800-237-6242

International Sports Science Association, Santa Barbara, CA
800-892-4772

National Academy of Sports Medicine, Calabasas, CA
800-460-6276

National Strength and Conditioning Association, Colorado
Springs, CO • 800-815-6826

YMCA, Chicago, IL • 800-872-9622

EQUIPMENT MANUFACTURERS

Concept rowers, concept2.com

Cybex, cybexintl.com

Freemotion, freemotionfitness.com

Hammer Strength

Lifestride

Nautilus, nautilus.com

Nordic Track, nordictrack.com

Paramount, paramountfitness.com

True, truefitness.com

Universal, universalgymequipment.com

FITNESS TIP: After a great day of nutrition and exercises, we still need a third part: proper recovery.

ENDURANCE TRAINING METHODS

30/30, consists of a single set of 30 exercises done in 30 minutes with no rest periods

Basic circuits, combination of high-intensity aerobics and resistance training designed to be easy to follow

Cardio circuits, high-intensity aerobics using various pieces of Cardio equipment with little or no rest periods

Hi reps, using over 20 reps per set

Isometric training, strength training in which the joint angle and muscle length do not change during contraction

Resistance training circuits, high-intensity aerobics using various types of resistance exercises with little or no rest periods

Slo-mo plyometric training, using slow motion movements in conjunction with plyometric exercises

Slo-mo reps, taking five or more seconds per rep

Speed-Agility-Quickness drills

Supersets, alternating two exercises for the same muscle group, taking as little rest as possible between each set

FATTEST CITIES

Houston

Philadelphia

Detroit

Memphis

Chicago

Dallas

New Orleans

New York

Las Vegas

San Antonio

Reference: About.com, "The 25 Fittest and Fattest Cities in America," losangeles.about.com ©2005.

FITTEST CITIES

Colorado Springs

Minneapolis

Albuquerque

Denver

Portland

Virginia Beach

Seattle

Honolulu

San Francisco

Milwaukee

Reference: "The Fittest and Fattest Cities in America," *Men's Fitness*, mensfitness.com/cityrankings/462, ©2008.

FITNESS BASICS

Be reactive and proactive

Improve all components of fitness, including strength, endurance, balance, and flexibility

Include proper nutrition

Include proper psyche

Include proper recovery periods (see

Keep routines progressive and integrated

Keep routines varied

Target all muscles

Train functionally

Use proper form

FITNESS TIP: The more intuitive one is, the more productive and progressive will be the training.

FITNESS BENEFITS GENERAL

Improved balance

Improved cardiac health

Improved coordination

Improved functionality

Improved overall health

Improved posture

Improved sex life

Improved sleep

Improved sports performance

Increased productivity at home, work, etc.

FITNESS TIP: Beware of absolutes in fitness and nutrition. As individuals we are affected differently by stress, environment and general living and playing. Find what works for you!

FITNESS BENEFITS PHYSICAL

Improved joint stability

Increased endurance

Increased flexibility

Increased musculature

Increased power

Increased range of motion

Increased strength

Reduced/maintenance of body fat

Reshaped body/body composition changes

Toned musculature

FITNESS TIP: Consider combining two of fitness modalities for fun and variety, eg, Cardio yoga, Cardio core, Spin/Weights, etc.

FITNESS BENEFITS PHYSIOLOGICAL

Decreased resting heart rate

Improved hormonal function

Increased aerobic capacity; cardio respiratory function

Increased energy

Lowered Cholesterol level

Lowered Triglyceride level; Improved lipid profile

Maintenance of bone health

Moderated and lowered blood pressure

Reduction or elimination of medication

Rehabilitation of mind and body

FITNESS TIP: The ACSM recommends 3–5 days per week of cardio for about 30–60 minutes.

FITNESS COMPONENTS

Agility

Balance

Body composition (percent fat and lean)

Coordination

Endurance (slow-motion reps, isolation exercises, cardiovascular, high reps, supersets, circuit training, multi-sets)

Flexibility (static, active, myofascial, PNF, yoga, etc)

Power, Plyometrics, Olympic exercises

Reaction time

Speed, e.g. time in the 100-meter dash

Strength, including dynamic training and isometric training

> **FITNESS TIP:** Focus training on the areas of your fitness that are more challenging. Minimalize time spent of those areas that are less challenging.

FITNESS MOVEMENTS

Boxing drills

Cardiovascular

Lunge

Pull

Push

Self-myofascial release

Squat

Trunk extension

Trunk flexion

Trunk twist

Note: Movement Assessments are basic movements from which poor biomechanics or compromised joints and muscles may be noticed.

FITNESS DISCIPLINES

Aquatics

Balance training

Cardiovascular training

Flexibility

Functional training

Indoor cycling and step class

Pilates

Resistance training

Tai Chi or Qigong

Yoga

FITNESS TIP: Meditation is a great way to improve health, find peace and understanding and relax.

FITNESS ROUTINES KEYS

Basic movements include squat, lunge, ab crunch, ab twist, arm push, and arm pull

Enjoy and appreciate exercise

Follow body composition, not body weight.

Have fun

Include rotation in exercises and stretches

Reduce your stress levels as work, home, etc

Remember, moderation rules

Take steps more frequently

Train low back as well as abdominals

Use variety

FITNESS TIP: Variety is the key to continued fitness success. Change routines, disciplines and all parts of your workouts as much as possible.

FITNESS CHALLENGES

Board balancing on spherical base

Boxing circuits

Disk squat and twists with eyes closed

Loaded box jumps

Loaded one-leg Romanian deadlifts

Loaded Sun salutation (ie, squat thrust/Burpee)

Negative/loaded dip and chinup

Stability ball hyperextensions throwing medicine ball

Stability ball side one-leg one-arm side plank isometric

Stepmill loaded running/treadmill shuttle running

> **FITNESS TIP:** Loaded plyometrics such as box jumps should be done infrequently to avoid injury.

FITNESS TRENDS BECOMING MORE POPULAR

Aerial yoga

Barre classes

Body weight training

Bokwa

Core training (not Ab training)

Functional training

Group training

High-Intensity Interval Training

Hot yoga

More yoga styles

Obstacle course training

Online training (group via website)

Virtual training (personally via webcam)

FITNESS TIP: Ashtanga, which uses these branches, means eight-limbed as described by Patanjali.

FITNESS TRENDS BECOMING LESS POPULAR

Ab classes

Bikram

Cardio machines

Cross Fit

Fad diets

P90X and other DVD systems

Pilates

Pole classes

Spinning

Weight training

Zumba

FITNESS TIP: Only commit to that which I have time and skill to accomplish completely and well (know when to say no).

GROUP EXERCISE MODALITIES

Combo classes

Dance-based classes

Equipment-based cardio

Inline skating

NIA

Pilates

Ramping

Rebounding

Slide training

Sports conditioning

Tai Chi

Yoga

Reference: Methods of Group Exercise Instruction, www.exrx, December 2012.

GROUP EXERCISE TYPES

Abs, a class that focuses on core training

Body sculpting, program using weight, flexibility, and endurance training without creating bulk

Circuit, a combination of high-intensity aerobics and resistance training

Indoor cycling, an aerobic exercise performed on stationary bike with music

Kickboxing/Boxing

Mat Science, a class that focuses on floor core training

Pilates, a method of physical and mental exercise involving stretches and breathing to strengthen the abdominal core

Step, a low-impact aerobics class that involves stepping up and down on adjustable platforms

Stretching

Yoga, a combination of breathing exercises, physical postures, and meditation

GYM BAG ESSENTIALS

Cap, visor, hair ties

Shorts

Shower shoes

Socks

Sunglasses

Toiletries

Towels

T-shirt

Water

Workout gloves

FITNESS TIP: Safe limited exposure to the sun, air and earth is vital for our health. Get outside once a day for 20 minutes.

YOUR VIRTUAL GYM BAG

Balance disk or Bosu ball

Comfortable clothing

Device with internet or phone service

Myoball or myoroller

Quality thick mat for both fitness and yoga

Resistant bands and dumbbells

Skype or other videoconferencing software

Stability ball

Water and Towel

Well lit, comfortable surrounding

FITNESS TIP: One of the most important tools for fitness is the myoball, good for pain relief, myofascial therapy, range of motion, flexibility and more.

INJURY TREATMENT

Acupuncture and/or reflexology

Compression, and Elevation

Contrast therapy

Heat (sauna, steam, hot tub etc.)

Massage

Physical therapy

R.I.C.E., a treatment method for soft tissue injury, which is an acronym for Rest, Ice, Compression, Elevation

Stretch

Take a break from exercises, up to one week

Visualization to speed healing

Work other joints

Reference: *Exercise Standards and Guidelines Reference Manual,* ©1995 Aerobics and Fitness Association of America, Sherman Oaks, CA.

JUDGING RESULTS

Are you more functional?

Are you sleeping better?

Do you deal with stress better?

Do you feel better?

Do you have more energy?

Do you look better?

Do your clothes fit better?

Is your body mass index (BMI) better?

Is your confidence higher?

Is your waist-to-hip ratio better?

Note: Stay off the scale!

MARTIAL ARTS TYPES

Aikido, a Japanese martial art employing principles similar to judo

Capoeira, an Afro-Brazilian art form that combines elements of martial arts, games, music, and dance

Hapkido, a dynamic and eclectic Korean martial art

Jeet Kune Do, a martial art, which means the "way of the intercepting fist," developed by Bruce Lee

Judo, a Japanese sport adapted from jujitsu similar to wrestling

Jujitsu, a method of self-defense without weapons that was developed in China and Japan

Karate, a Japanese martial arts style featuring strikes

Kickboxing, a group class combining kicking and boxing

Kung Fu, refers to the many diverse Chinese martial arts

Tae Kwon Do, a Korean martial art similar to karate

MOVING TO NEXT LEVEL

Add a sport

Add Cycling

Add Running

Attend a fitness workshop/certification

Add webcam training

Change gyms

Change your routine

Find a workout partner

Hire a Personal Trainer

Hire a second trainer

Train progressively

FITNESS TIP: Working out with others allows for fun, progressive ideas, variety and experimentation. Embrace what others have learned.

OVERTRAINING SYMPTOMS BY THOMPSON

Amenorrhea

Anemia

Atypical changes in recovery heart rate

Atypical changes in resting heart rate

Constant soreness leading to pain

Decrease in lifting performance

Decrease in strength

Fatigue

Muscle tears

Stress related injuries

FITNESS TIP: Your rising resting heart rate and its variances is a great indicator of health or disease.

OVERTRAINING SYMPTOMS BY WEIDER

Appetite loss

Chronic fatigue

Deterioration of ability to concentrate

Elevated AM blood pressure

Elevated AM pulse rate

Insomnia

Irritability

Lack of enthusiasm for workouts

Motor coordination deterioration

Persistent sore muscles/joints

Reference: *Ultimate Bodybuilding,* Joe Weider with Bill Reynolds, ©1989, NTC/Contemporary Publishing Group, Inc.

PHYSIOLOGICAL ASSESSMENTS

Blood Pressure

Body Composition

Cholesterol

Core assessment (situp/crunch)

Pull assessment (pullup/two-arm hang)

Pulse

Push assessment (pushup/modified pushup)

Shoulder stretch behind back

Sit and reach

VO2 Max, Maximum ability of the body to transport and utilize oxygen to the muscles

FITNESS TIP: Along with core muscular use and control, breath awareness, use and improvements (VO2 Max), leads to other areas of fitness progressing.

PERSONAL WORKOUT ESSENTIALS

Comfortable and breathable attire

Confidence

Gym etiquette

Head phones/iPod®

Medical alert bracelets

Proper footwear

Respect

Towel

Water

Workout gloves

Note: A swimming pool is a fantastic amenity at a gym or your home.

PERSONAL TRAINER ATTRIBUTES

Adaptable

Attentive and able to communicate

Fit

Good listener who answers questions

Optimistic, positive attitude

Professional

Punctual and reliable

Qualified and certified

Understands individual needs

Works from a body, mind, spirit basis

FITNESS TIP: Having more than one trainer or changing trainers occasionally is a healthy way to stay fit and learn about your body and mind.

PUBLIC GYM ESSENTIALS

Adjustable benches

Balance equipment

Cardiovascular equipment

Dumbbells and barbells

Group exercise programs

Medicine balls

Resistance bands

Resistance machines

Squat/power rack

Stability balls

FITNESS TIP: Stabilizing properly and well on stability balls leads to a stronger core for excellence in other fitness areas.

SAFETY BASICS

Use spotter as necessary

Wear proper footwear

Stay focused/alert

Know your limits and recovery periods

Reduce repetitious activities, use variety

Control your movements

Wash hands regularly

Wipe off equipment after use

Ask gym to purchase an Automated External Defibrillator

Beware of pools of sweat on floor

FITNESS TIP: Keeping a journal is a great way to find what works for you individually; what exercises, which disciplines, what foods, etc.

TRAINING ERRORS

Incomplete range of motion

Lack of Assessment/long term goals

Lack of focus and specificity

Lack of/too short warm-up

Minimal variety

Overtraining

Poor form

Too fast reps

Too much weight

Undertraining/too little intensity

FITNESS TIP: Proper breathing along with form is key to training properly and progressing.

TOP HEALTH RISK FACTORS

Cigarette smoking

Diabetes mellitus

Diagnosed high blood pressure

Family history of coronary disease or other atherosclerotic disease in parents/siblings prior to age 55

High cholesterol

High Resting HR

High triglyceride and/or abnormal

High-density lipoprotein ration

Obese/Overweight

Poor eating habits

Sedentary lifestyle

Reference: *Exercise Standards and Guidelines Reference Manual,* ©1995 Aerobics and Fitness Associations of America, Sherman Oaks, CA.

TOP FITNESS BOOKS

ACMS Personal Training Manual

Body Learning, 2nd Ed., Gelb

Core Performance, Mark Verstegen

Fitness For Dummies, 3rd Ed.

Hatha Yoga Illustrated, Kirk

Prescription for Nutritional Healing, Balch

Science of Stretching, M. J. Alter

Stretching, Bob Anderson

The Complete Book of Abs, K Brungandt,

The Fitness Book of Lists, Thompson

The Gray's Anatomy, Lippincott

The New Encyclopedia of Modern Bodybuilding, Schwarzenegger

The Pilates Body, Siler

The Power of Ashtanga Yoga, MacGregor

Three-Dimensional Treatment for Scoliosis, Lehnert-Schroth

Virtual Personal Training Manual, Thompson

TOP HEALTH BOOKS

Body Learning, Michael J Gelb, ©1994, Henry Holt

Feng Shui, Symbols of Good Fortune, Lillian Too, ©2007, Konsep

Hatha Yoga Illustrated, Martin Kirk, Brooke Book, Daniel DiRuro, ©2006

Parkinson's Disease, The Art of Moving, John Argue, ©2000, New Harbinger Publications, Inc, Bolinas, CA

Prescription for Nutritional Healing, Phyllis A. Balch, Penguin Group

Step-by-step Tai Chi, Master Lam Chuen, ©1994

Stretching, Bob Anderson, ©2000, Shelter

The Pilates Body, Brooke Siler, ©2000

The Power of Ashtanga Yoga, Kino MacGregor, ©2013

Three Dimensional Treatment for Scoliosis, Christa Lehnert-Schroth, ©2007

TOP MAGAZINES

Best Life, bestlifeonline.com

Fitness Rx for Women, fitnessrxmag.com

Fitness Rx, fitnessrxformen.com

Health, health.com

Men's Health, menshealth.com

MMI, emusclemag.com

Muscle and Fitness, muscleandfitness.com

Shape, shape.com

Women's Health, womenshealthmag.com

Yoga Journal, yogajournal.com

FITNESS TIP: Want to train with a friend or family member who lives across the country? Consider Webcam training, linking two or more clients to train live at the same time. A great way to stay in touch and get fit.

TOP HEALTH CLUBS

24 Hour Fitness, 24hourfitness.com

Bally Total Fitness, ballyfitness.com

Crunch, crunch.com

Fitness USA, fitnessus.com

Gold's Gym, goldsgym.com

LA Fitness, lafitness.com

Powerhouse, powerhousegym.com

The Sports Club/LA, thesportsclubl.com

Wellbridge, wellbridge.com

World Gym, worldgym.com

Reference: Top 10 Cardio exercises, top10links.com, ©2009.

TOP VIDEOS

Buns of Steel

Donna Richardson

Insanity® series

Karen Voight

Kathy Smith

P90x® series

RIP 60® series

Step Reebok

The Firm

Yoga Journal

FITNESS TIP: The more variety a video fitness program has, the better chance for success.

TOP WEBSITES

ACSM, acsm.org

Aerobics and Fitness Associations of America, afaa.com

Core Performance, coreperformance.com

eFitness, efitness.com

ExRx, exrx.net/Exercise.html

Performance Workout, performanceworkouts.com

Physical Genius, physicalgenius.com

primuswe.com/fitnesspartner

PT on the net, ptonthenet.com

The Fitness Jumpsite,

VirtuFit, VirtuFit.net

WebMD, aolsvhealth.webmd.aol.com/home

FITNESS TIP: ExRx has a detailed list of various muscles and their actions, important to understand how fitness movements affect our bodies and minds.

VIRTUFIT® OFFERINGS

Ashtanga yoga

Aquatic training

Core training

Flexibility

Functional

Group classes

Group personal training

Hatha yoga

Meditation

Personal training

Power yoga

Qigong

Rehabilitation

Spinning

Vinyasa yoga

Note: Go to www.virtufit.net for details.

WAYS TO AVOID TRAUMA

Allow proper recovery time

Always warm up prior to working out

Do not overdo it

Listen to your body

Protect your knees, use proper leg form

Remember RICE (Rest, Ice, Compression, Elevation)
and use when appropriate

Start out slowly

Wear proper, quality, comfortable foot ware

Reference: *The Only 127 Things You Need: A Guide to Life's Essentials,* Donna Wilkinson, Penguin Group, New York, ©2008.

WORKOUTS WHEN SHORT ON TIME

Basic circuits, combination of high-intensity aerobics and resistance training designed to be easy to follow

Descending sets, beginning with a lower rep weight and moving to a higher rep weight with little or no rest

High intensity sets

Interval training, repetitions of high-speed / intensity work followed by periods of rest or low activity

Pyramiding, doing first set with light weight for more reps, increasing the weight and finally decreasing the reps again

Same day AM/PM workouts

Sequences sets, adding one exercise every circuit without a rest period; up to 10 circuits

Shortened rest period, reducing or eliminating the rest period

Split system, split the body parts into two or three sessions and work out two or three times per week

Supersets, alternating two exercises for the same muscle group, taking as little rest as possible between each set

CHAPTER 8

Nutrition & Mindfulness

NUTRITION is the selection of foods and preparation of foods, and their ingestion to be assimilated by the body. By practicing a healthy diet, many of the known health issues can be avoided. (http://en.wikipedia.org/wiki/Nutrition)

MINDFULNESS is the practice of maintaining a nonjudgmental state of heightened or complete awareness of one's thoughts, emotions, or experiences on a moment-to-moment basis. (www.merriam-webster.com/dictionary/mindful)

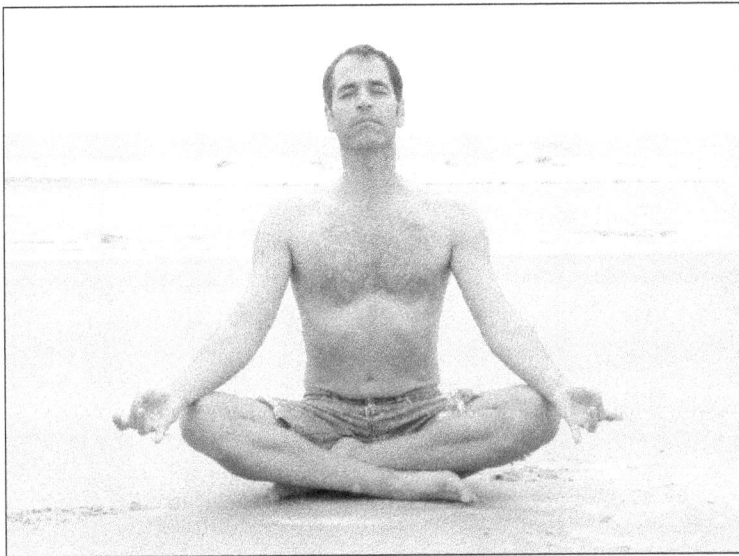

Bring health to your body, mind, and spirit.

ATTRIBUTES OF A QUALIFIED THERAPIST

Aquatic training

Balance & stability training

Basic strength & flexibility training

Core training (knowledge of yoga, pilates, tai chi & mat science)

Functional training (knowledge of integrated functional and dynamic functional training)

Mental training integrated into workout

Parkinson/Neuropathy background

Progressive and understand variety

Unilateral training

FITNESS TIP: As important is that therapy and fitness should be *Fun*. Therefore as Captain Jean-Luc Picard would say, "Make it so."

BODY SYMMETRY TRAINING

Alternating cable exercises

Asymmetric loading with two loads, heavier load on weaker side (Unequal loading)

Asymmetric loading with weaker side loaded, stronger side no load

Cable exercises

Dumbbell exercises

Train weak side first

Train weak side more often

Unilateral exercises

Weak side one-leg stance drills

Weak side Speed-Agility-Quickness drills

Note: Strength, flexibility, and balance usually vary from right to left sides. Train accordingly.

COMMON MOVEMENT PATTERNS

Gait pattern

Pull pattern

Push pattern

Squat pattern

Trunk extension

Trunk flexion

Trunk rotation

Reference: *Muscle Mechanics*, 2nd Ed., Everett Aaberg, Human Kinetics, Lower Mitcham, South Australia, ©2006

FITNESS TIP: Worthwhile books include *The Men's Health Home Workout Bible*, Lou Schuler and Michael Mejia, ©2002, Rodale, Inc., and *Men's Health: The Book of Muscle-World's Most Authoritative Guide to Building Your Body*, Schuler and King, Rodale, Inc.

COMMON POSTURAL IMBALANCES

Excess lumbar curve

Hyper extended knees

Pronated foot

Rounded upper back

Shortened/contracted hamstring

Shortened/contracted iliopsoas

Supinated foot

Upper cross syndrome

Weak abdominals

Note: Numbers 1–3 can be part of lower cross syndrome.

Reference: *Exercise Standards and Guidelines Reference Manual,* ©1995 Aerobics and Fitness Associations of America, Sherman Oaks, CA.

DAILY WONDERS

Drink ACV daily

Eat veggies daily

Exercise daily

Go barefoot daily

In sun daily

In water daily (tub, pool, ocean)

Meditate & pranayama daily

Practice yoga daily

Smile daily

Walk daily

FITNESS TIP: ACV (Apple Cider vinegar) has many uses aside from nutritional. Find out all the wonders of this product.

EATING HEALTHIER

Eat like a tourist in Greece

If you can't grow it, don't eat it

Read the back of the box first

The crunchier, the better

A frozen berry beats a fresh doughnut

You can't replace real ice cream

There's no fruit in "fruit flavor"

If it's not around, you can't eat it

Table your meals

Judge food by its cover

Cake's just not that into you

Don't drink dessert

Make sure you can ID the animal

Fuel up in the morning, not at night

Don't buy food where you buy tires

Work for your dinner

Your hips are not a fridge

Watching Top Chef isn't cooking

Cut yourself a break!

Source: www.self.com/body/food/2009/06/20-ways-to-eat-healthier

ESSENTIAL FOOD

Calcium sources

Fish, poultry and eggs

Fruits

Healthful oils (plant oils like olive oil or flaxseed oil)

Legumes

Nuts

Seeds

Vegetables

Whole grains

FITNESS TIPS: Most if not all minerals must come from food sources, not supplements. Many supplemental minerals are not absorbed or assimilated properly in the human body.

ESSENTIAL NUTRIENTS

Carbs

Fats

Minerals

Protein

Vitamins

Water

Reference: *The Only 127 Things You Need: A Guide to Life's Essentials*, Donna Wilkinson, Penguin Group, New York, ©2008.

EXERCISING YOUR BRAIN

Read

Meditate

Make Lists

Travel

Practice Neurobics

Play Word Games

Start an Intellectually Stimulating Conversation

Exercise

Switch Hands

Note: The brain's growth continues into adulthood. According to the Alzheimer's Association, engaging your brain builds a reserve of brain cells and connections and helps keep the brain healthier throughout aging. Completing daily brain exercises ensures you are utilizing one of your most important organs and staying mentally fit.

Source: www.ehow.com/list_6923554_10-ways-exercise-brain.html

FITNESS BENEFITS PSYCHOLOGICAL

Conquer challenges

Enjoy life

Feel better

Have fun

Improve socialization

Increase self-esteem, self-confidence

Look good

Maintain cognitive function

Reduce and relieve depression

Reduce and relieve anxiety

FITNESS TIP: The best easiest way to maintain overall health is to exercise the mind, spirit and body *at the same time.*

FITNESS MOTIVATORS

Begin a sport

Change clubs or trainers

Change workout days or times

Find a training buddy

Join a club or team

Set goals, both long and short-term

Take a week off from training

Train for an event

Train outdoors

Use head phones or watch TV during workout

FITNESS TIP: Socialization is important for health. Taking classes and having workout buddies is paramount.

FUN THINGS AUTHOR DOES

Drink tea in stainless steel or glass mugs

Put drinking water in glass containers (try using kombucha bottles)

Exercise my mind via brain gym each day

Exercise my body with variety each day (key term 'variety')

Finish eating when I am content, not when food is all gone (leftovers for next meal)

Go to bed at first sign of tiredness (sometimes that means 8 pm)

Make shakes/drinks with blender (but not with juicer, there's a difference)

Meditate

Take daily digestive enzymes (eg, kombucha, sea greens, probiotics, etc.)

Wake up without an alarm clock (I don't even have a clock in my bedroom)

GUIDE FOR POSITIVE THINKING

Consider the Consequences of Negativity

Contribute to the Community

Create a Daily Gratitude List

Establish and Work Toward Goals

Offer Compliments to Others

Practice Self-Care

Read Positive and Inspirational Material

Recognize and Replace Negative Thoughts

Spend Time with Positive People

Take Responsibility for Your Behavior

Reference: www.lifehack.org/articles/communication/10-tips-make-positive-thinking-easy.html, June 2014.

GYM ETIQUETTE

Carry a towel

Clean machines after use

Keep noise level low

Maintain control of weights and equipment

Replace used equipment

Respect other's space and be attentive

Share machines and equipment with others

Stay out of mirror-view of others

Use cologne and perfume sparingly, if at all

Wash hands regularly

FITNESS TIP: Exercising our eyes is important but often overlooked. Research ways to keep eyes healthy for life.

KEEPING EGO IN CHECK

Claiming our 'undesirable' parts as parts of ourselves that have lost their 'song'.

Contemplating deeply the meaning of the great truth: "Nothing can ever be truly obsolete."

Living a surrendered life that knows that the folly of others should be observed (but not engaged) as the mirrors of areas within ourselves where we need to express the song of self.

Releasing resentment against the pace of life. Our resentment indicates that ego wishes to keep control.

Relinquishing all need to define ourselves and to be understood.

Ruthlessly eliminating the focus on what is not the way we want it to be—this only increases the illusion of lack.

Reference: www.handbookforhealers.com/six-ways-to-eliminate-ego/, July 2014

KEYS TO POSITIVE THINKING

Action expresses priorities

Be the change

Find yourself in the service of others

Have a sense of humor

Learn as if you'll live forever

Our greatness is being able to remake ourselves

What you think you become

Where there is love there is life

Your health is your real wealth

Your life is your message

Reference: http://positivemed.com/2012/12/28/10-ways-to-improve-your-life/, July 2014.

MEDITATION BENEFITS PHYSIOLOGICAL

It lowers oxygen consumption.

It decreases respiratory rate.

It increases blood flow and slows the heart rate.

Increases exercise tolerance.

Leads to a deeper level of physical relaxation.

Good for people with high blood pressure.

Reduces anxiety attacks by lowering the levels of blood lactate.

Decreases muscle tension

Helps in chronic diseases like allergies, arthritis etc.

Reduces Pre-menstrual Syndrome symptoms.

Helps in post-operative healing.

Enhances the immune system.

Reduces activity of viruses and emotional distress

Enhances energy, strength and vigor.

Helps with weight loss

Reduction of free radicals, less tissue damage

Higher skin resistance

Drop in cholesterol levels, lowers risk of cardiovascular disease.

Improved flow of air to the lungs resulting in easier breathing.

Decreases the aging process

Source: www.ineedmotivation.com/blog/2008/05/100-benefits-of-meditation/

MEDITATION BENEFITS PSYCHOLOGICAL

Builds self-confidence.

Increases serotonin level, influences mood and behavior.

Resolve phobias & fears

Helps control own thoughts

Helps with focus & concentration

Increase creativity

Increased brain wave coherence.

Improved learning ability and memory.

Increased feelings of vitality and rejuvenation.

Increased emotional stability.

Improved relationships

Mind ages at slower rate

Easier to remove bad habits

Develops intuition

Increased Productivity

Improved relations at home & at work

Able to see the larger picture in a given situation

Helps ignore petty issues

Increased ability to solve complex problems

Purifies your character

Source: www.ineedmotivation.com/blog/2008/05/100-benefits-of-meditation/

MEDITATION BENEFITS SPIRITUAL

Helps keep things in perspective

Provides peace of mind, happiness

Helps you discover your purpose

Increased self-actualization.

Increased compassion

Growing wisdom

Deeper understanding of yourself and others

Brings body, mind, spirit in harmony

Deeper Level of spiritual relaxation

Increased acceptance of oneself

Helps learn forgiveness

Changes attitude toward life

Creates a deeper relationship with your God

Attain enlightenment

Greater inner-directedness

Helps living in the present moment

Creates a widening, deepening capacity for love

Discovery of the power and consciousness beyond the ego

Experience an inner sense of "Assurance or Knowingness"

Experience a sense of "Oneness"

Source: www.ineedmotivation.com/blog/2008/05/100-benefits-of-meditation/

MEDITATION TYPES

Walking Meditation.

Writing Meditation.

Eating Meditation.

Chakra Meditation

Chanting Meditation.

Music Meditation.

Koan Meditation.

Body Awareness Meditation.

Breath Awareness Meditation.

Light/ Flame/Object Meditation.

Note: All of these types of meditation are designed to bring your focus and awareness to the present moment. Being mindful during your day can provide you with many benefits. Don't discount it just because one type of meditation hasn't worked for you. There are many more types that you might try.

Source: http://hubpages.com/hub/10-Different-Types-of-Meditation-to-Try

NUTRITION BASICS

Avoid extreme diets, no-fat, low-carb, etc.

Eat a variety of healthy foods

Eat breakfast

Eat every 3 or 4 hours, small meals consisting of carbs-protein-fats

Eat in moderation

Eliminate chemicals, additives, artificial ingredients, etc.

Focus on whole foods as main food sources

Hydrate daily, but remember, you can drink too much water

Reduce or eliminate trans-fatty acids

Take multi-vitamin/mineral per health practitioner, powder or liquid preferred

Note: Seek organic produce when purchasing your plant foods.

POPULAR MANTRAS

aum (pronounced om or oom)

Aum Namah Shivaya

Aum Namo Narayanaya

Aum Shri Ganeshaya Namah

Aum Kalikayai Namah

Namo Arihantânam

Namo Siddhânam

Namo Âyariyânam

Namo Uvajjhâyanam

Namo Loe Savva Sahûnam

Om Namo Narayanaya

Om Namo Bhagavate Vasudevaya

Om Sri Ram Jai Ram Jai Jai Ram

Ram Nam

Tat Twam Asi

Aham Brahma Asmi

Source: http://mindbluff.com/mantra.htm

POSTURE BASICS

Keep car seat and office chair ergonomically sound

Keep computer area ergonomically sound

Keep purse weight below five pounds and alternate shoulders. Alternate which arm holds children.

Keep wallet slender and remove when seated, alternate pockets

Sleep with arms below head level on a mattress with proper firmness

Stretch hamstrings/lumbars for those who are seated for prolonged periods

Stretch pectorals/deltoids for those who frequently hold arms forward without support (hair stylists, physical therapists, drivers, etc.)

Use a head set when on phone

Use a step for support especially those who stand for prolonged periods of time (nurses, waitresses)

Use proper neutral spine/pelvis throughout day

FITNESS TIP: Stand as often as possible.

PRESERVING NUTRIENTS

Choose produce in bright and deep colors

Eat fresh produce within a few days

Only buy what you'll consume in a few days

Remove moldy or damages pieces

Store most produce in refrigerator

Store produce in separate containers

Wash all produce before eating, but not until you are ready to eat them

When cooking, use light, quick methods

When fresh is not an option, freeze produce or buy frozen produce

When possible, eat the peels and skins

Reference: *The Only 127 Things You Need: A Guide to Life's Essentials*, Donna Wilkinson, Penguin Group, New York, ©2008.

PSYCHOLOGY OF FITNESS

Be confident

Focus/concentrate

Identify weaknesses and improve

Leave ego at door

Listen to body signals

Make fitness a lifestyle

Meditate

Think about the mind-muscle link

Think positively

Visualize muscle targeted

FITNESS TIP: Yoga is the basis of many common disciplines, including pilates, ballet, stretching, etc.

RAISING YOUR CONSCIOUSNESS

Boost your brain power and functioning

Take full control of your lifestyle

Choose empowering beliefs

Avoid physical fighting and abuse

Be aware and accepting of your emotions

Speak compassionately

Think positive, act positive, be positive

Develop a deep relationship

Identify with your soul

See perceived faults as a "mirror image"

Expand your horizons

Face your deepest fears

Use powerful incantations.

Practice positive affirmations

Be aware of your state of consciousness

Set a positive example for others

Guide others interested in raising their consciousness

Share your unique insight and wisdom

Gain wisdom from others

Keep your ego in check

Source: www.themindfulword.org/2012/20-ways-become-more-conscious/#7vSAmW5OuhdiHQY6.99

RELAXATION SONGS

Celtic Spa

May It Be – Enya

Spa – Duduk Meditation Spa Music

December – George Winston

Serenity – Serenity Spa Music

Caverna Magica – Andreas Vollenweider

Armenian Duduk and Relaxing Ocean Waves – Spa Music

Piano Ecstasy – Relaxation Piano

Cristofori's Dream – David Lanz

Bamboo Flute Wellness – Asian Zen Spa Music Meditation

Source: www.meditationrelaxclub.com/top-10-relaxing-music-playlist-best-relaxation-songs/

TOP ANIMAL PROTEIN SOURCES

Free range eggs

Free range poultry (eg, chicken. Turkey)

Grass feed red meat (eg, beef, buffalo)

Mahi mahi

Organic plain yogurt

Scallops

Shrimp

Tilapia

Wild salmon/tuna fish

Note: Seek organic, non-hormone, wild, low-mercury, free-range, grass-fed when purchasing your protein foods.

TOP PLANT PROTEIN SOURCES

Beans

Blue-green algae

Dark leafy greens

Lentils

Nuts (eg, Almond, Cashew)

Quinoa

Seeds (eg, Hemp, Sunflower)

Spirulina and Chlorella

Sprouts

Tempeh

FITNESS TIPS: Protein sources generally occur naturally with healthy fats. Stay clear of fat-free or low-fat protein sources.

VISUALIZATION OF GOALS

Ask yourself what you want

Envision a specific act

Imagine big

Literally make it visual

Rehearse in your head

Review often

Surround yourself with similar dreamers

Think success

Verbalize your goals

Write in down

FITNESS TIP: Manifestation can occur naturally during meditation.

WAYS TO LEAVE YOUR LOVE HANDLES

Add natural colors to your nutrition

Change your routines

Choose whole foods

Eliminate toxic thoughts and behavior

Exercise during commercials

Order an appetizer as your main course

Park farthest in lot

Use smaller portions or plates

Use the stairs

Walk on bridge inclines

Reference: "50 Ways to Leave Your Love Handles," Accent, *Palm Beach Post*, January 2, 2008.

WAYS TO DESTRESS

Creative Expression

Cut Back On Caffeine

Exercise Regularly.

Get Massage

Get More Rest

Get Outside

Get Up A Half Hour Earlier

Listen to Music

Practice Yoga

Take a hot bath.

Reference: www.genpink.com/10-ways-to-de-stress/, June 2014

FITNESS TIP: Allow yoga to lead to meditation.

WORST THINGS YOU CAN DO FOR YOUR HEALTH

Drinking heavily

Eating processed food

Forgoing sunscreen

Having unsafe sex

Leading a sedentary lifestyle

Not flossing

Over medicating

Overuse of antibiotics

Skipping health practitioner's visit

Smoking

Stressing out

Reference: "Worst Things You Can Do for Your Health, 11 Worst Health Hazards," Laura Colarusso, aol body, www.aol.com, March 2008 .

CHAPTER 9

Fitness Quotes & Proverbs

Fitness takes work and determination, knowledge and regularity. Along the way it is important to keep a sense of humor, smile at the impasses and learn from the challenges. Allow these actual client conversation and modified proverbs put a smile on your beautiful face.

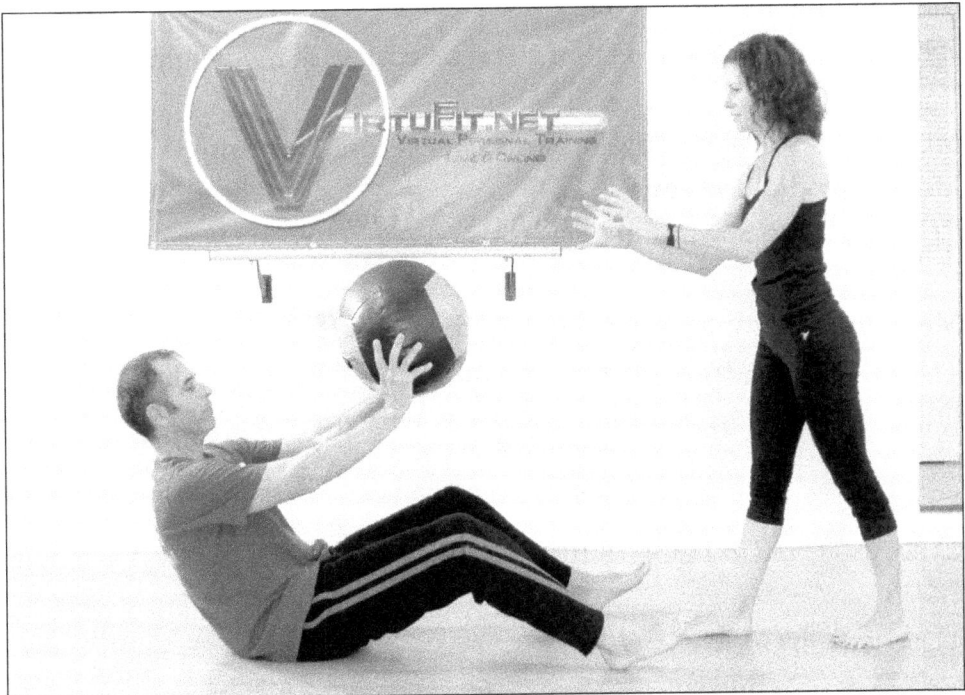

Medicine ball situps and throw

HUMOROUS CLIENT CONVERSATIONS

CLIENT: "I can't breathe!"
ME: "Breathing is overrated."

Silence....
ME: "Why did you stop?"
CLIENT: "I heard someone somewhere say 'Stop'."

CLIENT: "This exercise is EASY!'
ME: "Then we need not do it again."
CLIENT: "Oh." (defeated)

CLIENT: "I HATE this exercise!"
ME: "Then we need to do it more often."
CLIENT: "Oh." (defeated)

ME: "Situp tall."
5'4" MALE CLIENT: ". . . Is that a crack because of my height!?"

ME: "S–" (as in slow down), Same client stops exercising
ME: "Why did you stop?"
CLIENT: "Any 'S' word means Stop."

ME: "How many days a week would you like to train?"
CLIENT: "Three. Train me hard Monday and Wednesday, but Friday take it easy; Saturday I have sex with my wife."

ME: "...9...10..."
CLIENT: "THAT'S 14, NOT 10!"

CLIENT: "Oh God!"
ME: "Yes my child?"

HUMOROUS CLIENT QUOTES

"Am I supposed to feel a pulse in my ears?"

"Are the quads in my arms here?"

"But I need my kickstand." (when asked to lift arm and leg in table-top pose)

"Can I buy you with food?"

"Could you show me…?"

"Do you make other clients do this?"

"Do you think I threw up because I ate a Big Mac and fries before the workout?"

"Does this exercise make my butt look big?"

"Don't ever ask me to do that again."

"Eeek!" (mouse-like shriek while doing plank)

"El diablo!"

HUMOROUS CLIENT QUOTES (Cont.)

"Everything is creeky today!"

"Girls shouldn't have to do that!"

"Have you been holding back on me?" (said by patriarch of family when realizing his wife and two adult children had vomited during my sessions, but he had not)

"How dare you take away my training wheels." (when asked to lift foot while balancing)

"Huh?... balance on my chins?" (I had said shins)

"I brought my massage shoes." (translation: I wore sandals so I can't work out today)

"I can't do that, I left my reading glasses at home."

"I can't work out, this music sucks."

"I don't skip."

HUMOROUS CLIENT QUOTES (Cont.)

"I feel like a wooden soldier." (text received about being sore after first workout)

"I forgot my sports bra, can we skip that?"

"I hate all these!" (exercises)

"I just got fired." (when client was told I couldn't train him Saturday mornings anymore)

"I knew I should have worn underwear today!"

"I left my moxie at home."

"I sprained my eyes just now."

"I would rather not sweat, can we work out still?"

"I injured my rotary cup once."

"I'm calling my mom." (said by 68-year-old client)

"I'm too old for that!"

"If I do that, I'll fart for sure."

"Is that really an exercise?"

"Is this supposed to be hard?"

HUMOROUS CLIENT QUOTES (Cont.)

"Is that my traperzoids?"

"It'd be easier if I told you what doesn't hurt!"

"Jews don't do that."

"My armpits are shaking."

"My hair hurts."

"My last trainer said I don't need to do lunges, they're for girls."

"Never!"

"No thanks, didn't you know, white guys can't jump!"

"No!"

"Oh that exercise is for young people!"

"Oh, Jesus, Mary & Joseph!"

"Oh, my other left leg."

"Ooh, so that means I don't ever have to stretch!"

"Sorry, I didn't bring a jock strap."

HUMOROUS CLIENT QUOTES (Cont.)

"Ok, Ok, the safe is behind the painting in the bedroom…"

"That hurts sooo good."

"That's not comfortable for my…man parts."

"That's nothing my gladiator abs can't perform!"

"The KGB could have used you!"

"There's a muscle there?"

"They call my butt tank-tard glutes"

"This exercise makes me feel like a kid."

"This is Stupid!"

"Today, can we exercise through osmosis?"

"What's the name of this torture."

"What's a burpee?"

"When did you retired from the Spanish Inquisition?"

HUMOROUS CLIENT QUOTES (Cont.)

"Where do you dream up this sh**?"

"Where did you learn to count?!"

"Why?"

"You can do anything you want to me, but I cannot bleed, vomit, or pass out."

"You found a way to stop a woman talking; train them so hard they can't."

"You put the 'S' in S and M."

"You train me like I'm in shape!"

"Your training reminds me of those Chinese torture boxes . . . you know."

"You would have excelled helping with the Spanish Inquisition!"

. . . burp!

. . . fart!

HUMOROUS PROVERBS

A body is only as strong as its weakest link.

A journey of a thousand miles starts with a single lunge.

A kingdom is lost for want of a TRX.

A lifter's work is never done.

A little inactivity is a dangerous thing.

A loaded Olympic bar makes no noise.

A man is known by the P90X he keeps.

A man's gym is his castle.

A medball in the hand is worth two in the bush.

A roll-out gathers no moss.

A watched muscle never peaks.

A yoga pose is worth a thousand words.

Ab work loves company.

All's well that exercises well.

An organic apple a day keeps the doctor away.

Before criticizing a man, walk a mile.

Bike while the iron is hot.

Don't put all your dumbbells in one basket.

Early to tread and early to exercise, makes a man healthy, wealthy and wise.

Fitness is the better part of valor.

Fitness makes the heart grow stronger.

Fitness makes the world go around.

Give a man a dumbbell and you exercise him for a day; teach a man to exercise and you give him health for a lifetime.

He who sedentates is lost.

Health speaks louder than words.

Health wasn't built in a day

Home is where the squat rack is

I came, I saw, I burpee'd

I stress, therefore I exercise.

If a pose is worth doing, it is worth doing well.

If all else fails, try jump squats.

If at first you don't succeed; lat fly, lat fly again.

If in doubt, go lift.

If the shoe fits, do butt kickers.

If you can't take the heat, get out of the gym.

If you fail to exercise, then you exercise to fail.

If you snooze you lose (. . . your muscles)

If you want something done right, crunch it yourself.

It ain't over till the calf muscle stings.

It's better to have jump-squatted and puked than never to have jump-squatted at all.

Jump squats are like war, easy to start, hard to end, impossible to forget.

Learn to walk before you run (then learn to sprint~!)

Life is just a bowl of dumbbells

Life is like a box of expert trainers' workouts. You never know what you're gonna get.

Life is what you do while you're waiting for a treadmill to open.

Lift and let lift.

Lift and the world lifts with you. Whine and you whine alone.

Look after the dumbbells and the pounds will look after themselves.

Loose hips sink ships.

Luck favors the fit.

Lunge softly, carry a big stick.

Lunge twice, squat once.

Man is truly himself when he's toned.

No strain, no gain.

Nothing adventured, nothing gained.

One good rep deserves another.

Our greatest glory is not in never squatting, but in rising every time we squat.

People who live in glass houses shouldn't throw weights.

Physique and ye shall find.

Practice what you preach(er curl).

Repetition is the mother of hypertrophy.

Show a man a squat, he's healthy for a day; teach a man form, he's healthy for the rest of his life.

Skiing is believing.

Split or get off the pot.

Sticks and stones may break my bones but crunches will never hurt me.

The bends justify the genes.

The bicep is always bigger on the other guy.

The burpee is greater than its parts.

The core shall set you free.

The dumbbell swings both ways.

The longest mile is the last mile of marathon.

The only stupid exercise is the one that is not performed.

The truth is in the spine.

There's always a flexion before an extension.

There's more than one way to chin a bar.

There's no accounting for waist

There's no arguing with pair of bicep guns.

There's no medball like an old medball.

There's no such thing as a free lunge.

Think before you oblique.

Time flies when you're flexing guns.

'Tis better to have lifted and lost than to have never lifted at all.

To jump squat is human; to vomit, divine.

Too many crunches and not enough back extensions.

Two sleds are better than one.

Use it or lose it.

Variety is the spice of the gym

Waist not, want not.

Wellness is bliss.

Wellness talks, disease walks

What you sow is what you rep.

When in om, do as the omans do.

When one core contracts, another core relaxes.

When the going gets tough, the tough get another rep.

When the mat is away, the abs will decay.

Where there is a will, there is a weight.

Glossary

Airplane: arms out to sides, 90 degrees in frontal plane.

Body weight: only using the body, no machine, balls or weights.

Bridge: supine, hips lifted, for most exercises this is an isometric, see Hip lift.

Bridge on SB: face up on back or ball, knees bent, hips elevated on a stability ball.

Burpees: an exercise also called squat thrusts, modeled after yoga's sun salutation

Calf raise: lifting heel(s) of feet.

Circuit: moving from one exercise or station to another with minimal rest.

Close stance, narrow stance: feet closer than hips width.

Contralateral: moving or using (balance) opposite arm and leg simultaneously.

Dip position: Supported on a bench or chair, hips lifted supported by hands with legs out front.

Down dog: Downward facing dog pose.

Dumbbell Hi plank: hi plank holding dumbbells in hands.

Face me: turn so that client faces trainer (camera).

Flex: indicates stretches or rehab exercises organized for a particular purpose or for a class.

Front raise: lifting straight-arms from hips out front to shoulder level.

Hi lunge: Lunge with arms overhead.

Hi plank: pushup position, on hands and toes.

Hip Lift: bridge position, lifting hips up and down.

Interval: alternating high- and low-intensities movements, with periodic rest periods.

Isometric: holding a position, a pose.

Lat: latissimus dorsi, a large upper back muscle.

Lateral: movement away from the body to the side.

Low lunge: lunge with hands on floor by front foot.

Low plank: plank, on forearms and toes.

Lunge: standing with one foot in front of other, with both knees close to 90 degrees, back knee near floor.

maha mundra: seated single bent knee hands to foot, flat spine yoga pose.

Myocore: A session combining myowork and core exercises.

Myowork: Use of myoball and myoroller for stretching, pain reduction, range of motion and myofascial release.

Myoball: Small foam ball used for muscle stretch and work.

Myoroller: Foam cylinder used for muscle stretch and work.

Neutral grip: palms facing each other.

Open boat: supine with arms and leg straight and lifted slightly.

Paulina: supine legs in air, hip lift exercise.

Plyometric: exercises that involve jumping, throwing/catching and/or rapid movements.

Prone: lying face down.

Rear fly: lifting straight-arms out to side to shoulder level while bent over (not to rear).

Reverse tabletop: supine position on hands and feet, knees bent, hips elevated. Also crab.

savasana: supine yoga pose, corpse.

Scorpion: an exercise lying prone, alternating leg lift across other leg.

S-I Joint: the pelvic Sacroiliac joint.

Side lunge: Stepping laterally and lowering.

Side raise: lifting straight-arms from hips out to side to shoulder level.

Slash (/): this generally designates "and" and is placed between two exercises. One performs both exercises back to back, one rep of one exercise, one rep of the other, repeatedly.

Split stance: one foot forward.

Squat: lowering from standing to sitting position and returning.

Superdog: prone tabletop, positioned on hands and knees, usually lifting contralateral limbs.

Superman/Supergirl: Lying prone (face down), arms outstretched to front.

Supine: lying face up.

Swimmers: superman usually with contralateral arm and leg raise.

Tabletop: Either supine position on hands and feet, hips elevated, knees bent or reverse tabletop prone position on hands and knees. Also table pose.

Turn to side: turn so that trainer see client from the side (camera to side).

Up dog: Upward facing dog pose.

VPT: Virtual Personal Training or Virtual Personal Trainer, i.e. personal training and class taught via webcam.

Wall sit: sitting against wall or back on ball against wall in a squat position, thighs parallel, back vertical, hands on hips.

Wide stance: feet wider than hips width.

About the Author

Marc D. Thompson delved into writing and genealogy at a very early age. He wrote stories, poems, lyrics and family history books. Marc went on to write and research in high school and college, earning a BS degree from Moravian College. He has presented genealogical lectures and authored over ten family history volumes. Marc's other published works include *The Fitness Book of Lists, Virtual Personal Training Manual, Fitness Quotes of Humorous Inspiration* and a poetry compilation, He currently pens a genealogy blog at google blogger and wrote a monthly genealogy column for Atlantic Avenue Magazine. He is a member of the Association of Professional Genealogists, founded a PA Genealogy Society and was the County Coordinator of the Chatham Co, GA USGenweb site. Marc believes in what he calls Creatalytical Thinking: The fusion of creativity and analysis to view life more fully and fulfill his place in this world. Writing now for over four decades, Marc has been influenced by science, art and his relationships, and yet marvels at the cosmically-driven direction he receives from energy around him.

www.ingramcontent.com/pod-product-compliance
Lightning Source LLC
Chambersburg PA
CBHW082350270326
41935CB00013B/1567